SURVIVING MRSA

Learn how to Protect Yourself

by

Dr Joseph Parazoo

Dr Joseph Parazoo

Copyright: 2009 by Dr Joseph Parazoo

All rights reserved. No part of this book may be reproduced, stored in a retrieval system, or transmitted in any form or by any means without the prior written permission of the publishers, except by a reviewer who may quote brief passages in a review to be printed in a newspaper, magazine, or journal.

ISBN: 1449517145
EAN-13: 9781449517144.
Printed by CreateSpace
an Amazon.com company
Scotts Valley, CA

www.joeparazoo.com

Printed in the United States of America

Surviving MRSA

Dr Joseph Parazoo

Dedication

It is your right and duty to be responsible for your own health and well being. I know that this statement is contradictory to what most people believe and what the Doctors tell you.

I dedicate this book to those of you that take on this task, and to those of you that take your spiritual journeys serious.

Surviving MRSA

Dr Joseph Parazoo

Acknowledgments

First, I thank God, our Great Creator of the Universe, for providing the love, strength, and guidance to overcome this horrific experience; and then for all of the great and wonderful experiences that followed.

Second, I thank my wife Kim. For if it wasn't for her strength, I don't know how I would have made it.

I would also like to thank all the dedicated people in the medical field for all of their work.

Surviving MRSA

Dr Joseph Parazoo

Table of Contents

Disclaimer		.....	Page 12
Introduction		.....	Page 14
Chapter One	The Flu	.....	Page 16
Chapter Two	Protect Yourself	.....	Page 28
Chapter Three	Confused	.....	Page 32
Chapter Four	Septic Shock	.....	Page 40
Chapter Five	Going Downhill	.....	Page 44
Chapter Six	Fournier's Gangrene	.....	Page 54
Chapter Seven	Reading the Signs	.....	Page 56
Chapter Eight	The Symptoms	.....	Page 64
Chapter Nine	How it Spreads	.....	Page 68
Chapter Ten	Skills at Work	.....	Page 72
Chapter Eleven	Strep A	.....	Page 80
Chapter Twelve	Squabbles	.....	Page 84
Chapter Thirteen	Strep B	.....	Page 88
Chapter Fourteen	Progress	.....	Page 90
Chapter Fifteen	Crossed Wires	.....	Page 100
Chapter Sixteen	Dreaming	.....	Page 108
Chapter Seventeen	Necrotizing Fasciitis	.....	Page 116
Chapter Eighteen	Fears of the Dark	.....	Page 122
Chapter Nineteen	MRSA	.....	Page 130
Chapter Twenty	Skin Grafts	.....	Page 138
Chapter Twenty One	Treatment	.....	Page 150
Chapter Twenty Two	Preventing	.....	Page 156
Chapter Twenty Three	Rehabilitation	.....	Page 162
Chapter Twenty Four	Transformation	.....	Page 174
References		.....	Page 180
About Author		.....	Page 186

Surviving MRSA

Dr Joseph Parazoo

Formal Disclaimer

This disclaimer is to provide myself as Author of this book some legal protection:

- The Author is not a medical professional so any claims he makes are not backed up by any type of professionally accepted scientific evidence or formal training on his part.

- The Author is not an herbalist or pharmacologist so is not claiming that his suggestions in using herbs are based on any specialized expertise on his part.

Caution and review of suggested supplements with experts is always recommended to make sure the individual doesn't have any medical side effects.

- The Author is not a Minister or Priest in any formal religious tradition so does not claim any special expert knowledge in those traditions.

- Any information or pictures in this book which the Author did not write may have been copied and modified from publicly available sources on the internet.

Surviving MRSA

Dr Joseph Parazoo

Introduction

It begins with a minor injury, usually on an extremity. You complain about having the flu, and go about your normal routine.

Wounds of any kind will hurt, but in this case the pain is excruciating. Fever sets in, and an unusual redness develops around the area of injury and rapidly moves away from the initial site. By the next day, the redness has turned a strange blue color.

The skin begins to blister horribly, the blister containing sickly yellowish to bluish fluid. Some of these blisters may burst, causing an eruption of foul-smelling pus and loss of large amounts of blood. The pain at this point is severe, almost intolerable.

Sometimes the pain is so bad that you no longer feel it. By day four, it is obvious that gangrene has set in. At the hospital, surgeons plunge into a desperate, exhausting battle against the disease, fervently hacking away flesh that becomes rotten almost as fast as scalpels can cut it away. The prognosis is very poor, and the struggle for life continues until death or disfigurement comes—or maybe both.

This is a tale of a vicious disease that has a preference for human flesh, an appetite that surpasses the worst of nightmares.

However, this is not like a nasty Hollywood horror movie, that might keep you up all night in terrified fascination. This one is made by Mother Nature, and is very, very real…

This is a story inspired by one such…real case.

Surviving MRSA

Dr Joseph Parazoo

Chapter One
The Flu

In a small town near the Oregon coast, the year 2005 had just started to unfold itself. Sheridan, with a population of just over five thousand, nestled in the heart of the Willamette Valley, where the soil is rich, and the days are pleasant. It is small and quiet, yet not too far from all of the amenities.

The day was just another warm day in January. It was about 11:30 in the morning, when the phone rang. *"Hello."* It was my wife, Kim. Just one of the many calls I had received over the years, during her lunch break. She was feeling a little under the weather. Complaining about the flu.

"If you feel that bad, why don't you just come home?"

The electric-green Mustang convertible pulled into the driveway of the two-story older home. The house was sitting on a double lot, on a peaceful and quiet street. It was in need of some paint, but the yard was well groomed. It looked older than the birth date of 1949, for it had been a rental all of its life.

She walked between the rose bushes that lined the sidewalk. The two biggest ones were about four feet tall and probably two and a half feet wide. They were yellow, her favorite color.

I could tell that she didn't feel very good, when I opened the door, and greeted her with a kiss. *"I really feel like shit. I'm going to go to bed."* Working at the local casino, there is always "some bug" floating around.

Surviving MRSA

Group A streptococcus normally live in people's throats and can spread in the community from person to person. Often, up to fifteen percent of people may "carry" the bug without knowing and without suffering any illness. Group A streptococcus spreads very easily in conditions where people are housed together in close quarters.

Group A streptococcus also can live on the skin, particularly where the skin is damaged by conditions such as eczema, as well as on any other mucous surface of the body. It cannot survive for very long away from the human body.

In the twenty-seven years of our marriage, I've never known her to be that sick. *"No problem. I'll fix you some soup."* I put together a nice arrangement, and took the tray into the bedroom. *"I fixed you some chicken soup. And here is some juice... Can I get you anything else?"*

"No, thank you," she said. She was looking a little pale.

"Get some rest now," I said as I left the room.

Often, NF occurs in otherwise healthy, active individuals. No major trauma is necessary. In fact, the condition often occurs following minor trauma, or even a bruise or abrasion. Perhaps the most troubling and frightening aspect of NF is its remarkable ability to **mimic minor afflictions—which fools both the patient and the doctor.**

NF often mimics common post-operative symptoms such as severe pain, inflammation, fever and nausea, which also thwarts a timely diagnosis. Education and awareness by the general public as well as the medical community in recognizing symptoms is critical to saving lives.

Dr Joseph Parazoo

Afternoon rolls around, I hear, *"Honey, could you come here. I would like to show you something."* She showed me a spot on her right buttock cheek that must have hurt really bad.

I saw a baseball-sized reddish area that was slightly swollen. There was a dime-sized whitish area near the center, with a small hole. The part that bothered me was the grayish-black edges of that hole. *"Let me clean it up a little, there is a little blood,"* I told her as I walked toward the bathroom.

I swallowed hard. I'm not really sure what it was that I was feeling, but I didn't like it. I had this sick feeling in my stomach. An intolerable sense of fear. Fear of loss. After gathering a few cleaning supplies, I washed my hands and walked back into the bedroom.

I started to clean the area and noticed that the hole was a little larger than I thought. The grayish-black stuff that I saw was meat. I was actually washing her raw flesh.

As I washed the outer part, where the redness was, this yellowish stuff that reminded me of honey started to come out of the wound. That was followed by some really dark blood, and the worst odor that I had ever smelled.

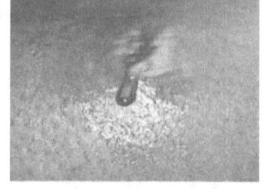

"Doesn't this hurt?" I asked as I continued to clean up the area. She said that it didn't hurt, even though she knew that she should be feeling some pain. *"We need to go to the hospital. I have done as much as I can."*

I didn't have to say anything; she already knew that it must be serious. McMinnville was sixteen miles away, and

Surviving MRSA

had the closest hospital. With a population of almost thirty thousand, it was the home of the ever-popular Linfield College.

I tried not to let my thoughts of worry show. Kim remained quiet, thinking to herself, *What the hell is going on? I have had the flu before, but, never this bad. Why do I have this dreaded feeling I might die? God, Don't let me die.... I haven't seen enough sunsets, with my husband..... I want to see my son, James, get married and be happy.... I need to spend more time with my daughter, Kathy, and the grand kids.*

These are supposed to be doctors; why aren't they doing anything? I spent the next few minutes steaming, as the anger was really building up inside of me. They seemed to be more interested in accusing us of things, than taking care of the problem. So far, they haven't ran any tests. They just look and guess at what might be going on. *"I could do that much."*

After a few more minutes that seemed like hours, another doctor came in. He had a better approach than the other guys. He introduced himself as Dr. General Surgeon and addressed me.

"I can understand why you are getting upset. You are worried about your wife. The thing you have to remember, is this is the first time any of us has seen your wife. We don't have any history. We are trying to figure out what the problem is before we decide what the best course is. Has anything like this happened before?"

"No," I replied. He was an older gentleman, somewhere in his sixties. His hair was thin and gray. He stood five foot ten, and supported a pot belly, yet he was not fat.

Dr. General Surgeon said, *"I want to run some blood tests, and take her into surgery. That wound has to be cleaned up to find out what is going on. Maybe the tests will reveal*

Dr Joseph Parazoo

some better answers. I don't expect that the surgery should take very long. It will take longer for the anesthesia to take effect. In order for me to ask Kim questions, I will be using a spinal." He turned around as he reached for the doorknob, and then said, *"I'll talk to you when I am through."*

NF is a rare bacterial infection that can destroy skin and the soft tissues beneath it, including fat and the tissue covering the muscles (fascia). These tissues often die rapidly. NF is very rare but serious. Many people who get NF are in good health prior to the infection.

They prepped her for the surgery and started to wheel her down the hallway. I kissed her and said, *"Don't worry, you are going to be all right.... Take care of her, Doc,"* I continued as the doors closed behind the moving bed.

Kim thought to herself, *There must really be something wrong, in order to have surgery. The last time that I had a spinal, I was able to go home with a baby.*

The bed was pushed through the doors. The overhead lights were bright, and filled the room. Four people were already in the room waiting. *"Ready? One, two, three, and move."* In one smooth move, the four pairs of hands slid the woman from the bed to the operating table.

The table was made of stainless steel, and sent a chill through her body. Before anything could happen, they rolled her on her side. The anesthesiologist took the needle and inserted between the third and fourth lumbar. After depressing the plunger, he removed the needle, and discarded it. Within moments, she was completely numb from the waist down. She was rolled one more time, until she was face down.

"Scalpel," he said as he walked into surgery position.

NF is a rare infection of the deeper layers of skin and subcutaneous tissues (fascia). Many types of bacteria can cause NF, of which Group A streptococcus is the most common cause.

It consists of one or more bacteria, that cut off the blood supply to a part of the body. From there, it **spreads very rapidly**.

This stuff is very tricky, because it likes to **live under the skin**. It can go undetected for some time as it "eats" up the soft tissue.

The following depicts general symptoms of NF as the disease advances....... Trauma (day zero): This trauma does not have to be major, like getting hit with a baseball bat, or a car accident; it could be as small as a bee sting, hemorrhoids, pimple, or ingrown hair. Discomfort in the general region of the trauma (day zero). Pain that is out of proportion with the injury. Influenza-like symptoms such as vomiting, diarrhea, dehydration, weakness, muscle pain, and fever. Swelling or sunburn-type redness in the general region of the injured area (day two).... Worsening of the condition. Less frequent urination.

When the infection is caused by the lightning-fast Group A Streptococcus bacteria, people can **go from perfectly healthy to death's door in a matter of days.**

Other cases of NF, caused by a mixed bag of bacteria, can be slower moving and less deadly. In all cases, however, prompt treatment is essential in this condition. It is one of the fastest-spreading infections known, so time is the most important factor in survival.

Dr Joseph Parazoo

After about an hour, I saw Kim being wheeled out into the hallway. Dr. General Surgeon said, *"I couldn't really find any major problems. But, since she has a fever, I want her to stay in the hospital for observation. I will look in on her tomorrow."* Within a few minutes, we were escorted to a semi-private room.

About six o'clock the next evening, Dr. General Surgeon walked in. *"How are we feeling today, Kim?"* he asked as he put on a pair of rubber gloves.
"I'm feeling okay," Kim said.
"Your fever has come down," he said as he looked at the clipboard. *"Would you roll over please?"* he asked as he lifted up her gown. He pressed around the area. *"There isn't much swelling."*
"What happened? I mean, what caused this?" I asked.
"There was a swelling of the subcutaneous tissue, caused by some internal pressure. Probably a pocket full of infection. This caused the discoloration of the skin. At some point, the pressure was too much, and it erupted," he replied as he removed the bandage from the wound.
"What is that subcutaneous tissue?" I asked.
"That is the soft tissue, including the fat that lies underneath the skin."
"How did the infection get there?" I asked

NF is a bacterial infection. This bacteria attacks the soft tissue and the fascia, which is a sheath of tissue covering the muscle. NF can occur in an extremity following a minor trauma, or after some other type of opportunity for the bacteria to enter the body such as surgery.

Surviving MRSA

"I don't know how it got there. She might have had a pimple, boil, or an ingrown hair...and somehow it got infected." He pulled the bloody piece of gauze from inside of the wound. *"I don't see any infection. Her blood pressure was fine. Her white count was normal. Her sugar level was only one thirty-five. With running a fever like she was, I wouldn't say that was a problem."* He placed another batch of gauze in the wound. *"I don't see why you can't go home."*
"Is there anything special we need to do?" I asked.
"No, not really. She should stay home for a few days and rest.... I'm sure she will be a little sore. I want to see you Monday or Tuesday, at the office." He handed me a business card.

The Lee Stark NF Foundation has this to say: Complications of infection, rather than representing an infection in themselves. Severe bacterial infection causes a multitude of effects in the body.
The body attempts to fight the infection, but sometimes the immune response is amplified to an abnormal degree. Harmful products can be released by different parts of the body's immune system (white blood cells, blood vessels, the liver) which lead in turn to fever, low blood pressure, and failure of several of the body's main organ systems.
This is known as "septic shock" and can occur in response to any bacterial infection which is severe. Products released by the bacteria themselves may also contribute to this cascade of events.
Bacteria like strep (and also Staphylococcus aureus) make a number of toxins which, on their own, can trigger a huge and potentially harmful inflammatory response in people.

Dr Joseph Parazoo

We weren't told what the problem was. To my knowledge, she hadn't seen the wound.

The doctor said that the wound wasn't very big. It looked pretty big to me. There was a hole you could put a fifty-cent piece in. But, I didn't know how deep it went. The area was still a color between pink and red. At least all of the grayish-black stuff was gone. I still could smell a foul odor.

Though the toxins them-selves also appear to cause a characteristic rash or redness ("erythema") which turns whitish if pressed ("blanching"). This is known as "toxic shock" and really represents a subset of "septic shock".

Group A streptococcal (strep) infections are caused by group A streptococcus, a bacterium responsible for a variety of health problems. These infections can range from a mild skin infection or sore throat to severe, life-threatening conditions such as toxic shock syndrome and NF.

Most people are familiar with strep throat, which along with minor skin infection, is the most common form of the disease. Health experts estimate that more than 10 million mild infections (throat and skin) like these occur every year.

I knew that Kim was sick. But, by the evening, she seemed to be acting "sickly." She did not really want to eat or drink anything. I noticed that the area of the redness grew, but at least it wasn't swollen much. It now went from her hip to about halfway down to her knee, on the back of her leg.

"Every time I put pressure on my leg, my knee hurts." I thought that she might have twisted it or something. I looked more closely at her knee. There wasn't any swelling that I

Surviving MRSA

could tell. She said that she didn't twist it or anything.

It was a dull pain, more like someone squeezing on the inside. She was running a little fever, but not too high. We both thought that she was still suffering from the flu, plus the added pain from the surgery. But, we found out later how wrong we could be.

She was in so much pain, and with the high fever, she had to struggle into the office. After the fact, I should have bypassed the doctor and gone straight to the hospital.

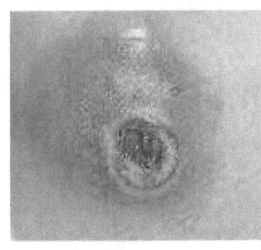

"Would you lean over this table, please," the doctor said as we entered the room. He lifted up her nightgown and took a look at the wound. With the scalpel in his hand, he started to cut away some of the gray flesh. Shortly after he started, he said, *"We need to put you in the hospital. Now!"*

"I don't want to go to the hospital," Kim said as she began to cry.

"I know you don't, honey. But we have to."

"I mean, I don't want to be bad enough that I have to go to the hospital." I understood actually what she meant. But there was absolutely nothing that I could do about it.

Dennis Stevens, MD, says: "STSS usually begins with a skin infection or an infected wound.. Within 48 hours of infection, the victim's blood pressure drops dangerously low, and she may experience dizziness, fever, labored breathing, confusion, rapid pulse and peeling skin rash."

Dr Joseph Parazoo

Surviving MRSA

Dr Joseph Parazoo

Chapter Two
Protect Yourself

**It's not the Flu that kills you,
it's the secondary infection (MRSA?)**

Why does this matter? Because in 1918, many of the deaths were not directly due to the influenza virus. Instead, they were caused by 'secondary' bacterial infections that ordinarily wouldn't have killed people:

Their findings are striking in the context of modern conceptions of the 1918 pandemic; the great majority of deaths could be attributed to secondary bacterial pneumonia caused by common respiratory pathogens, particularly pneumococci, group A streptococci, and staphylococci, and not to the virus itself.

Their conclusions are strengthened by the remarkable consistency in theme, if not details, displayed across the many studies reviewed and the inclusion in their review of not only gross pathologic findings but blood and lung tissue culture data. In only 4% of the more than 8000 cases reviewed was no bacterial super-infection documented.

The article also reports that K. pneumoniae was implicated in the deaths of these patients (although it was less frequent than the Gram-positives), along with other Gram-negatives, such as E. coli.

And if we can't treat these patients due to antibiotic resistance, the number of deaths which are kicked started by influenza, but ultimately due to bacterial infection, will be higher than anyone is currently thinking about.

A list of some of the most troublesome categories or

Surviving MRSA

species of streptococcus and the diseases for which they are well known includes:

Group A: strep throat, scarlet fever, rheumatic fever, impetigo, toxic streptococcal syndrome, streptococcal kidney disease, blood infections.

Group B: blood infections in newborns, meningitis, childhood fever.

Groups C, D, G, H, K: urinary tract infections, heart infections, meningitis, upper and lower respiratory tract infections

Streptococcus mutants: dental caries (cavities) Streptococcus pneumonia: Pneumonia, ear infections, meningitis, sinus infections.

There are more than **80 known types of Group A streptococcus, which can cause more than a dozen different illnesses.** Some of the more well-known Group A strep afflictions include upper respiratory disease such as strep throat and scarlet fever, skin disorders such as impetigo, and inflammatory diseases such as rheumatic fever or kidney disease.

Staph infections hit 12 million every year

With the dog days of summer and warm-weather sports in full swing, it's important to pay special attention to cuts, bruises and rashes that occur along with the fun. Staph — one of the most common skin infections in the United States — is responsible for 12 million to 14 million doctors' visits each year.

Close contact with others, sports that involve skin-to-skin contact, and warm, humid environments are a fertile breeding ground for staph infections. Staph bacteria can live

Dr Joseph Parazoo

harmlessly on many skin surfaces, especially around the nose, mouth, genitals and anus.

Basically speaking, strep in any form is easy to spread. It is a very common bacteria that lives in and on people.
So, in order to keep from the bacteria developing into something more serious, you have to take care of your wounds. You have to maintain a daily cleansing routine. You should eat a "healthy" diet, in order to keep your immune system in top condition.

The strep bacteria is spread through direct contact, and occasionally through coughing, kissing and other mucous swapping activities. You can be a carrier of strep without showing any symptoms.

Surviving MRSA

Dr Joseph Parazoo

Chapter Three
Confused

The doctor must have called ahead and made some preparations. When we walked through the doors, we bypassed the check-in desk. Kim was helped into in wheelchair and taken to an exam room. Within minutes, Kim was on a gurney.
"*Blood pressure ninety-six over sixty-eight,*" was the call of one nurse.
"*Pulse one hundred and regular.*" She reached for the electronic thermometer. Within seconds the thermometer beeped. As the nurse took it out of Kim's mouth, she read off,
"*Thirty-eight point one.*"
"*Let's get some bloods cooking. CBC, lytes, glucose STAT. Couple of extra tops for an SMA and tox screen,*" an intern barked out.
"*I can't get the needle in the vein, it's too small,*" the inexperienced phlebotomist responded as she continued to try and draw blood.
The anesthesiologist walked in and yelled at her, "*You can't be drawing blood from those veins. I need them for putting in the IV. Here, let me do it.*"
"*But I haven't drawn enough to run the tests,*" the nurse responded.
Just about that time Dr. General Surgeon. walked in and asked, "*Why don't you have her on oxygen? I told you she needs it. Can't you tell her breathing is labored?*"
One of the nurses grabbed the plastic mask. She placed it over Kim's mouth and nose. With the elastic strap

Surviving MRSA

holding it into place, the flow of oxygen started to flow.
Meanwhile, another nurse had the ER clipboard. She was using the cryptic code of medical shorthand. VSS for vital signs stable. PERRL for pupils equal, round, and reactive to light. The anesthesiologist was now trying to draw blood from her calf. Within minutes, she was "prepped" for surgery.
The basic test results showed up. *"Her blood sugar is over five hundred... Is she a diabetic?"* Dr. General Surgeon said as read off the information.
"No! Wouldn't we have said something before? Besides, you said last week that it wasn't a factor."
"Her white blood count is just over five thousand." I knew that the white blood cells were for fighting infection. I didn't know the values or what high or low meant. My assumption was, the higher the count, the more you are fighting an infection. I was escorted out to the waiting room. I thought to myself, *What the hell is going on? Why is she so sick?*

White blood cells are cells of the immune system, responsible for protecting the body from infection and malignancy. A white blood cell count (WBC) is ordered to check whether the number of white cells in the blood is abnormally high or abnormally low. Patients with a low WBC are at increased risk for infectious disease. The normal white blood cell count is between 4,500 and 10,000. A high level indicates an underlying problem that requires medical evaluation. It could indicate infection and tissue damage

I'm not a doctor but, according to that information, she was on the low side of normal. That information doesn't really tell me much more than I already knew. I guess that I would have to study more about that, in order to figure out

Dr Joseph Parazoo

what the values meant. As far as I am concerned, that is a minor thing, at this point. I knew that she had an infection…. Duh.

Just in case you didn't know: there are a lot of things that run through your mind in a time like this. Especially when you have no clue as to what is going on, or what they are doing. I won't mention any of the things that ran through my head, even if I did remember what they were. Two things that did trouble me (since he stressed them) were the blood sugar and the white blood count. To be honest, I just wanted her to be okay.

Time went by so slow as I paced many floors, waiting impatiently. I tried not to think about all of things that could be going on. I called our son, James, to let him know that I had to take his mother back to the hospital.

I tried to fill him in on the happenings of the day. When out of the corner of my eye, I saw the doctor strolling down the hallway. Looking at my watch, 7:30. When he was close enough, I asked, *"How is she, Doc?"*

"That's one strong lady you have there. I had to perform more debridement of the infected area."

"How much?"

"It was the size of a fifty-cent piece. Now it is about the size of a softball. She has staph. So I am going to keep her in intensive care tonight."

I knew that staph was short for staphylococcus, and that it was an infection. I really didn't know a lot more than that. *"Can I see her?"*

"Okay. Once she is in the room, I'll let you see her for a couple of minutes. You have to stay out of their way."

It seemed like hours, but within minutes, I was allowed to see Kim. I walked into the ICU, and saw Kim.

Surviving MRSA

The Group A Strep infection is most common with minor trauma. A mixed bacterial infection is often the cause after surgery. Group A Strep is the same bacteria that causes strep throat. However, there are various strains of the bacteria, some of which are more powerful than others. If the right set of conditions are present, this is when the NF occurs.

She just lay there, asleep. Just looking at her, with all of those tubes and machines hooked up to her, made my heart skip. I sure didn't like the feelings that were running through my body and mind. I reached out and grabbed Kim's hand. I knew she was asleep, but I swore she smiled. After holding her hand for a while, I was asked to leave. I kissed her good night, and told her that I would be back tomorrow. *"I love you, honey."*

"Her pressure is dropping."
"Can we draw some stat electrolytes? And hand me a blood gas syringe."

I don't think that I was in bed an hour, when the phone rang. *"Hello."*
"This is the Willamette Valley Medical Center. We are taking your wife back into surgery for another debridement. You don't have to come in, we just wanted you to know."

What kind of a person do they think I am? I know I can't do anything. But of course I want to be there. So, back to the hospital I go. It is about 1:00 in the morning by the time I get there.

"Your wife is already in the surgery. It will be some

Dr Joseph Parazoo

time before we hear anything."

The nurses didn't know anything. The doctor was busy. I couldn't talk to anyone that knows what is going on. As I paced the hospital hallways, I thought to myself, *What happened in such a short amount of time? Did that staph infection get worse? I sure wish that I knew something.* These, plus a lot more things continued to fill my head as I covered the floors of the hospital. I couldn't even get a cup of coffee.

Finally, about 2:00, I saw the doctor coming down the hallway. *"How is she? What's going on?"*

"Your wife is septicemic."

"What does that mean?"

"It means that she has a bad infection. And her body is full of toxin."

"What can be done about it?"

"We are doing everything that we can. We are giving her antibiotics. I also had to take a little more tissue from around the wound. There's nothing we can do now, but wait. Why don't you go home and get some rest. We are running more tests; I'll know more later."

Taken from Wikipedia (an internet encyclopedia):

In septicemic plague, there is bleeding into the skin and other organs, which creates black patches on the skin. There are bite-like bumps on the skin, commonly red and sometimes white in the center. Untreated septicemic plague is universally fatal, but early treatment with antibiotics reduces the mortality rate to between 4 and 15 percent. People who die from this form of plague often die on the same day symptoms first appear.

Surviving MRSA

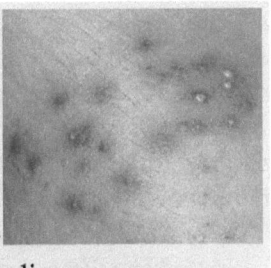

The "plague" appeared in three forms: bubonic, septicemic and pneumonic. The main characteristic of the septicemic plague was an infection of the blood. See also: Black Death—a plague in the 14th century that killed a third of the population in Europe. Many modern researchers have argued that the disease was more likely to have been viral and was spread by direct human contact. By the 20th century, the death rate is down to three percent of the population."

Oh, sure, my wife has staph infection.... and septicemic.... She has been in surgery twice within just a few hours... And you want me to "get some sleep" and not worry.... It is a lot easier to say than to do. I said to myself as he walked away.

During the Middle Ages, this plague was characterized by the appearance of petechiae; these were small, purplish, hemorrhagic spots on the skin. In extreme cases, the petechiae became almost black and spread until large areas of the body were afflicted by them.

So, what was this doctor trying to tell me? Was he trying to say that my wife had some kind of "plague"? I thought those were gone. Besides, where could she have caught it? I thought that "the plague" was some thing of the past. With all of the modern technology, I thought that it was wiped out. If she did have the plague, then she probably could die.

I located the nurse that was in charge of Kim and

Dr Joseph Parazoo

asked her what "septicemic" meant. She said, *"It's just a doctor's term that means that the body can't handle the amount of infection on its own. A better description would be 'septic shock.' So, it is better to keep the patient asleep and pump a lot of antibiotics in order to fight the infection."* I believed what she said, it made sense.

"Do you know how much tissue he had to remove?"

"The wound area is about the same size as it was. He went under the skin, and had to take a little tissue. The packing takes one of those four-inch rolls of gauze."

I might as well look up that "septic shock" that the nurse talked about.

Surviving MRSA

Dr Joseph Parazoo

Chapter Four
Septic Shock

The Lee Spark NF Foundation says: Septic and toxic shock are complications of infection, rather than representing an infection in themselves. Severe bacterial infection causes a multitude of effects in the body. The body attempts to fight the infection, but sometimes the immune response is amplified to an abnormal degree.

Harmful products can be released by different parts of the body's immune system (white blood cells, blood vessels, the liver) which lead in turn to fever, low blood pressure, and failure of several of the body's main organ systems. This is known as "septic shock" and can occur in response to any bacterial infection which is severe.

Products released by the bacteria themselves may also contribute to this cascade of events. Bacteria like strep (and also Staphylococcus aureus) make a number of toxins which, on their own, can trigger a huge and potentially harmful inflammatory response in people.

Group C and G strep's were not thought to be able to do this, but recently it was shown that some of these bacteria can actually make toxins similar to the group A strep.

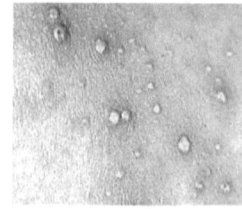
Though the toxins them-selves also appear to cause a characteristic rash or redness ("erythema") which turns whitish if pressed ("blanching"). This is known as "toxic shock" and really represents a subset of "septic shock".

Surviving MRSA

According to Dennis L. Stevens, PhD, MD, Professor of Medicine, University of Washington School of Medicine, Seattle, Washington:
Recently, severe invasive Group A Streptococcal (GAS) infections associated with shock and organ failure have been reported with increasing frequency, predominantly from North America and Europe.
These infections have been termed streptococcal toxic-shock syndrome (STSS). The complications of current GAS infections are severe; bacteremia associated with aggressive soft tissue infection, shock, adult respiratory distress syndrome and renal failure are common; **30% to 70% of patients die** in spite of aggressive modern treatments.
He continues by saying: Pain, the most common initial symptom of streptococcal TSS, is abrupt in onset and severe, and usually precedes tenderness or physical findings. The pain usually involves an extremity but may also mimic peritonitis, pelvic inflammatory disease, pneumonia, acute myocardial infarction, or pericarditis.
Twenty percent of patients have an influenza-like syndrome characterized by fever, chills, myalgia, nausea, vomiting, and diarrhea. Fever is the most common early sign, although hypothermia may be present in patients with shock. Confusion is present in 55% of patients, and in some, coma or combativeness is manifest. Eighty percent of patients have clinical signs of soft tissue infection, such as localized swelling and erythema, which in **70% of patients progressed to necrotizing fasciitis** or myositis and required surgical debridement, fasciotomy or amputation.
STSS, the disease usually begins with a skin infection or an infected wound.. Within forty-eight hours of infection, the victim's blood pressure drops dangerously low, and she

Dr Joseph Parazoo

may experience dizziness, fever, labored breathing, confusion, rapid pulse and peeling skin rash.

You can die within two or three days, unless treated with antibiotics and amputation of affected areas. But STSS is still a step down from the king of all strep infections: necrotizing fasciitis.

After reading the information from Dr. Stevens, it looks like she has a strep infection, and not a staph infection, or…maybe both. Was Dr. General Surgeon wrong in saying that she had staph? Or did she have both?

I sure didn't like that sentence that said *thirty to seventy percent of people with this "septic shock" die.*

Maybe it is a good thing that I wasn't more familiar with the term. I also didn't like the sentence about where *seventy percent of the people develop necrotizing fasciitis.*

Whatever that was, it sure didn't sound very good. I just wanted her to be okay. Even today, this information still brings a lump to my throat.

NF is a progressive, rapidly spreading, inflammatory infection located in the deep fascia, with secondary necrosis of the subcutaneous tissues. Because of the presence of gas-forming organisms, subcutaneous air is classically described in NF.

The speed of spread is directly proportional to the thickness of the subcutaneous layer. NF moves along the deep fascial plane. The overall morbidity and **mortality is seventy to eighty percent.**

Surviving MRSA

Dr Joseph Parazoo

Chapter Five
Going Downhill

I tried to get some sleep. However, there were a lot of things going on in my head. I admit, I was real worried.

"Her pressure is dropping."
"Get another IV started. Increase the amount of fluid. We have to get that pressure up." "Take her to OR three." The nurses scrambled around the bed, complying with the orders.
    Within minutes, she was wheeled into the operating room. Dr. General Surgeon was dressed in the green scrub suit, cap and mask. He pulled on a pair of rubber gloves as he approached the stainless-steel table.

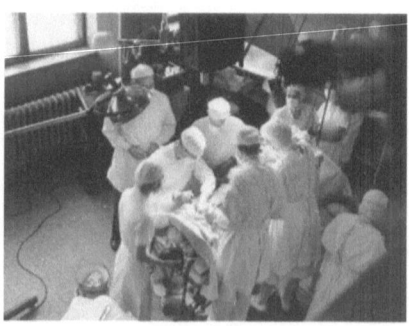

"*Pressure is stable,*" the anesthesiologist remarked.
"*Scalpel.*" The scrub nurse placed the scalpel in his hands.

    Finally it was four o'clock. Making sure that every-

Surviving MRSA

thing was set for the weekend, I got into the car, and headed for McMinnville. I don't really remember the drive from work to the hospital. I guess I just had too many things on my mind.

"Sorry, you can't see her now," was the response from the nurse when I asked to be buzzed into the intensive care unit.

"What's going on?"
"Your wife is in surgery."
"Why?.... What happened?"
"She is suffering from toxic shock... I'll let him know that you are here as soon as he is through."

Talk about a shock, and things running through your mind. To keep from being any more upset than I was, I walked down to the coffee shop in the lobby.

The 16-ounce mocha gave me a little energy as I paced the hallways. My mind was racing with many unfounded ideas of what might be happening. The air in the hospital started to feel stuffy and quite heavy. *"I best go outside."*

The jet was a Boeing 737. I was sitting in the aisle seat of row twenty-four. As soon as the seat belt clicked shut, I had the urge to look up. Walking down the aisle was this beautiful young woman. She stood five feet four, and was about 120 pounds. Her honey-colored hair was parted down the center. The feathered bangs were a nice accent to her shiny hair that grew to the middle of her back. *It sure would be nice, if she sat next to me. There is an empty seat,* I thought to myself.

To my surprise and delight, she stopped at my row. As she slid by me, I caught the scent of Wind Song, my favorite perfume. The three-hour flight was over in no time. That was the most comfortable conversation that I have ever had with a

Dr Joseph Parazoo

girl.

When she stood up to leave, she handed me her phone number and said, "If you are ever in Denver, look me up." It is hard to believe that was over twenty-five years ago. I remember it as if it were yesterday. It sure doesn't seem like it has been that long.

I walked back into the hospital and saw the doctor coming down the hallway. *"How is she? What's going on?"*
"She is a fighter, I have to say that for her. She is holding her own. We are doing everything we can. We're dealing with more than one bacteria. There must be five or six, and causing all kind of problems. This is beyond my expertise, and we are transferring her. We are calling around now, trying to locate a bed. We will let you know as soon as we know. This takes time. She is probably back in the room by now. Why don't you go see her."

It gets into the body, quickly reproduces, and gives off toxins and enzymes that destroy the soft tissue and fascia, which quickly becomes gangrenous (dead). This gangrenous tissue must be surgically removed to save the life of the patient. The bacteria also stealthily hides itself from the body's innate immune system, allowing it to spread rapidly along tissue planes.

NF causes excruciating pain, dangerously low blood pressure, confusion, high fever, and severe dehydration due to the toxins poisoning the body. Unfortunately, NF sometimes occurs beneath the skin with few symptoms to explain the victim's symptoms. This results in a great many cases of misdiagnoses.

Surviving MRSA

I made my way back to the intensive care unit. It took a few minutes, but finally I was let in to see Kim. She looked so helpless just lying there. She looked the same now as she did three surgeries ago.

A queasy feeling built up in my stomach. I didn't really know what caused it. I was at a loss as far as what was going on. At this point, the doctor had not really given me any "real" answers as to what was going on.

All he talked about was staph and bacteria. She had been on antibiotics, she had been in the doctor's care, three surgeries. Why can't they get it under control?

Finally, about ten o'clock, one of the staff doctors said, *"I found a spot at Emanuel. She can be moved in the morning. She is stable now. Why don't you go home and get some sleep. Be back about seven, we can go from there."*

The double swinging doors burst open as the bed was pushed through. The nurse flipped on the light switch as they entered the OR. The three bright lights instantly filled the room.

"One, two, three, and move." The four pair of hands smoothly moved the woman onto the stainless-steel operating table. The anesthesiologist turned on the machines and reconnected the leads. He moved into the normal position at the head of the patient. The scrub nurse took an inventory of tools as they lay on the tray.

Dr. General Surgeon was at the scrubbing sink, washing, when he thought to himself, *What is going on? At this moment all I can do is try and keep her alive.* After he completed his wash, he backed into the operating room.

He pulled on his gloves, while he approached the table. The normal assisting crew was already in place, and just waiting. *I can't let these thoughts cloud my judgment.* With

Dr Joseph Parazoo

scalpel in hand, he started to remove the gray, dead tissue from around the edges of the wound.

    I walked into the ICU, right at seven o'clock Saturday morning. *"Good morning. How is she this morning?"*
    "We tried to get a hold of you last night, but you weren't home. We had to take her back into surgery."
    I looked over at Kim, and I was almost speechless. She looked like a balloon, her whole body was swelled up. It almost seemed like she was a blimp, with all the wires and tubes plugged into her, as if to hold her down to earth.
    She had small tubes running along her face. They were clipped in her nose, providing oxygen. There was a stand beside her, with bags hanging from it. Each of the bags had medicine of some kind.
    Both of her wrists were bandaged and there was some black strip on her forehead. I tried to hold it back, but a tear rolled down my face. *"What the hell happened here last night? She was fine when I left."*
    The nurse responded, *"Calm down. The swelling is from all of the liquids that we are giving her. The walls of her blood vessels are weak, and the liquid is seeping into her body. This helps with her blood pressure; it is a little low. The vein in her wrist collapsed. So, we put one in the chest; it has several inlets. It makes things much easier too."*
    I walked over to Kim, bent down and kissed her. *"Hang in there, hon, everything is going to be all right."* Reaching for her hand, I noticed there was a solid black spot between her thumb and index figure. I asked, *"What is that thing?"*
    The anesthesiologist was taking a few readings, and replied with, *"That is a brain wave monitor. It keeps me informed of whether she is awake or not. With the amount of*

Surviving MRSA

pain she is in, I want to keep her asleep, so she doesn't feel it."

"That makes sense. Why are her wrists bandaged up like this?"

"When they were operating on the original spot, they noticed that the bacteria jumped there," the nurse replied.

"What do you mean...it jumped there? What kind of bacteria are we talking about?"

"She has gangrene."

As soon as I heard the word gangrene, my mind went elsewhere. I had heard of it before. You know, in the old westerns and war movies. After someone gets shot or something, they do not get medical treatment and get infected. Then they have to amputate.

But, she has been in the hospital for three days. Been taken care of, surgeries and antibiotics. How could she have gangrene?

According to the Mayo Clinic: Gangrene is the medical term for death of tissue (necrosis) in part of the body. It's a serious condition that requires immediate medical care. There are several types of gangrene. Symptoms depend on the location and cause. Treatment depends on the underlying cause. However, treatment can't revive dead tissue. Surgery or amputation often is needed to remove dead tissue.

"Actually it's called Fournier's Gangrene. This stuff has a mind of its own. It goes where it wants to," the nurse continued.

I'd never heard of this "Fournier's Gangrene." I wondered what it was. *"You mentioned operating on the other spot. What do you mean?"*

"They had to cut away some more at the original spot.

Dr Joseph Parazoo

Size wise, I guess almost the size of a softball. It crawled around to the inner part of her leg, toward the front."

"I never heard of anything like that."

"I know that you have been in touch with her mother. Call her; She needs to be out here."

"Why? What are you saying?"

"Your wife could lose her leg. And, if this stuff gets into her bloodstream, she could lose some of her organs. Or worse, she could die."

The more she talked, the more I could feel the pressure of the liquid. My eyesight was starting to get a little blurry. *"I thought we were getting transferred this morning."*

"The room we had lined up last night fell through. They are calling around to find another spot."

"I have to go for a little walk. I'll be back in a few minutes," I said as I headed for the door.

I located the first restroom. I hate to admit it, being a guy and everything, but as I was washing my hands, I just couldn't hold back any longer; I broke down and cried. My head was filled with questions and concerns.

After a few moments, I was able to compose myself. *"Maybe some milk will calm my stomach,"* I commented to myself.

"Can I have a 16-ounce mocha, please?" I asked the clerk as I walked towards the coffee shop. The automatic doors closed behind me as I reached for a cigarette. I don't really know how long I wandered around under the trees; it felt like only a couple of minutes.

I must have started to daydream. The brisk wind whistled through the trees, and rustled the few dry leaves across the ground. My mind was preoccupied; I didn't even notice the goose bumps that covered my arms.

Surviving MRSA

Kim laughed as she threw another handful of mud at me. I couldn't help but notice how cute she looked all covered with the dry mud. As I thought to myself, *Building this rock fireplace sure was fun, just being able to spend time together. It is times like these, that make this marriage.*

I have never been a religious person, and hardly ever pray. But I thought to myself, *I tried everything else..What could it hurt?*

"Dear God. You know that I haven't talked to you much. And I don't deserve it. But, I don't know what is going on, and I don't want her to die. If it is her time, take her now, so that she does not suffer. But, if it's not her time, please help her get through this. Amen."

Ring...Ring... "Hello. Mom, I have some bad news."
After the phone was silent, I walked back into the hospital. As the doors slid closed behind me, I headed in the direction of the coffee shop. "Can I have a 16-ounce mocha please?" I asked, not quite myself. My brain had so many things running through it, that I was walking in a fog.

After swigging about a quarter of the hot liquid, I dialed the phone. *Ring...Ring...* "Hello, Dad. I have some bad news." I am sure that he knew that, just by the tone in my voice. I was still rather dazed by the recent information.

I started to make my way down the hallway. Headed for the ICU.

"I've been looking for you. We have some good news."

"Kim is okay? And awake?"

"Sorry, it's not that good. We located another bed. In

Dr Joseph Parazoo

Providence. It will be ready by eleven o'clock this morning." I looked at my watch; it was 9:15.
"Where is Providence?"
"It's up in Portland. I'll give you a map. We have a lot of prep to do in order to get her ready. So, you might as well go home now. I'll ride up with her; she will be in good hands. The doctor that she will be seeing is one the best surgeons in the state."
Finally, maybe we can get some answers, I thought to myself as I drove home. How can someone be fine one minute, and be near death in the next? Why does she need another surgeon? Why did it take so long to find out what was going on? These questions plus a lot more were running through my head. I didn't want to spend the next few hours just thinking. I decided to find out what this "Fournier's Gangrene" was.

Surviving MRSA

Dr Joseph Parazoo

Chapter Six
Fournier's Gangrene

According to Thomas Santora, MD. Director of Regional Resource Trauma Center, Temple University Medical Center:

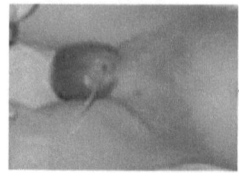

Fournier's Gangrene is a necrotizing infection that involves the soft tissues of the male genitalia.

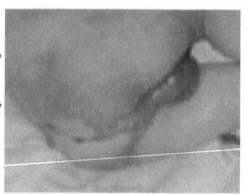

In modern-day vernacular, Fournier's Gangrene is a specific form of necrotizing fasciitis, a general term introduced in 1951 by Wilson to describe infection of soft tissue that involves the deep and superficial fascia, regardless of location. Modern day use of the term Fournier's Gangrene should be restricted to describe infections that primarily involve the genitalia.

The indiscriminate use of this eponym makes comparing the results of clinical series or defining a reliable occurrence rate difficult. In the 600 cases of Fournier's Gangrene discovered during a MEDLINE search dating back to 1996, 100 deaths occurred (16.5%). In the series that included more than 20 patients, the mortality rate ranged from 4-54%, with most studies reporting **mortality rates of 20- 30%.**

Surviving MRSA

Dr Joseph Parazoo

Chapter Seven
Reading the Signs

Beep... Beep... Beep... The ambulance backed up to the loading dock. The doors swung wide open as they pulled the stretcher out. *"What's the history?"* snapped the ER doctor.
"This is that transfer from Willamette Valley Medical." They wheeled the stretcher down the hallway, toward ICU.
"We've been expecting you."
"Ready? Watch that IV! One, two, three, and move!" was barked out. In one smooth transfer, four pairs of hands slid the woman from the ambulance stretcher onto the bed. Two of the nurses scrambled around the bed untangling IV lines, and connecting EKG wires to the cardiac monitor.
"Okay, let's get some bloods cooking. CBC, lytes, glucose STAT. Couple of extra red tops for SMA and tox screen."
"Her pressure is falling. Turn up that IV!" Within moments, the blood pressure was stable. About that time, she started to gasp for air. *"I'll put the airway in. Hand me the number seven ET tube."* The crash cart nurse passed him the laryngoscope and ripped open the ET tube packet. The doctor crouched down by the patient's head.
"Okay, let's do this." Tilting the head back, he slid the laryngoscope blade into the patient's throat. At once he identified the vocal cords. He slid the plastic endotracheal tube into place. The oxygen line was reconnected, and the machine turned on.

Surviving MRSA

Dr. Disease Buster walked over to the nurses' station, picked up the phone and dialed the lab. *Ring...*
"This is the lab, Rick speaking."
"When you run the chemistry panel on this transfer, make sure you test for electrolyte disturbances, glucose intolerance, and sepsis-induced metabolic disturbance."
"Yes, sir."
"I also want a complete blood cell count to assess the immunologic stress."
"Got it."
"Run an evaluation on the potential sepsis-induced thrombocytopenia. And I want a coagulation profile, containing prothrombin time, activated partial thromboplastin time, platelet count, fibrinogen level, to look for sepsis-induced coagulopathy."
"I'm on it," Rick replied as he hung the phone up.

Dr. Disease Buster was an intellectual man; he had the distinction of graduating at the top of his class. He was very interested in medicine, but not socially inclined. He would rather spend all of his free time in a library. He decided that he would specialize in infectious diseases. He liked the challenge of the hunt. He had a brilliant diagnostic mind. Dr. Disease Buster needed to make one more call. *Ring...*

"Radiology," was the response when the phone was picked up.
"I would like to run an ultrasonography on this transfer." This test can be used to detect fluid and/or gas within the soft tissues.
"What transfer is that?"
"The transfer from Willamette Valley Medical Center."
"I'll be there in ten."

The immunologist put a drop of blood onto the slide.

Dr Joseph Parazoo

He placed the stain under the clips, and turned on the light. He peered into the eyepiece, and adjusted the focus. This is an excellent tool in the detection of substances in a variety of diagnostic techniques. Standard applications of this include immunoblotting, ELISA and immunohistochemical staining of microscope slides.

The speed, accuracy and simplicity of such tests has led to the development of rapid techniques for the diagnosis of disease and microbes. It didn't take long to determine the blood type.

Dr. Disease Buster completed the pathologic evaluation. His hunches were right. We were dealing with necrosis of the superficial and deep fascial planes, fibrinoid coagulation of the nutrient arterioles, polymorphonuclear cell infiltration, and there were microorganisms identified within the involved tissues.

In others words; necrotizing fasciitis, (NECK-ro-tie-zing fashee- EYE-tiss) or flesh-eating bacteria.

Necrotizing fasciitis is a rare disease, that is what everyone has told me. The Office of Rare Diseases, of the National Institutes of Health, defines a "rare disease" as any disease that affects less than 200,000 people, throughout the entire United States, within a year. **See Chapter Seventeen.**

Ring... Ring.... "Hello."
"Hi, Kathy, hon. Your mother is in the hospital.... You should be here."

This stuff sounds like some scary shit. I sure hope they can get it under control. Looking at the above definition of Fournier's Gangrene, it still doesn't sound like they know what they are talking about.

Surviving MRSA

What makes me say that? My wife is not a male, for one reason. There is this phrase: "Fournier's Gangrene is a specific form of necrotizing fasciitis." Now what the hell is necrotizing fasciitis?

I was sure glad that James decided to drive. I don't remember much of the sixty-mile drive. My mind was so full of thoughts, that I was still in a fog. I must have been running completely on adrenalin. For the past three days, I'd been living on coffee and about six hours' sleep. We were on the freeway over half of that distance. It still took us almost an hour and a half to get there.

Everything passed me by in a blur, yet in slow motion. We walked through the main doors of this huge hospital, and caught sight of a bronze statue. The statue was of a nun named Mother Joseph. "That sure is a coincidence. This hospital is dedicated to one of our ancestors."

The statues and all of those stories are about Mother Joseph. Her real name was Esther Pariseau. She was born in Quebec, Canada, back in the 1800s. When she was young, she wanted to dedicate herself to a religious life and helping the poor.

Providence Health and Services, serving Washington, Oregon, California, Alaska and Montana, continues the caring traditions established by the intrepid pioneer sister and her colleagues 150 years ago. Mother Joseph's life has provided a wellspring of inspiration for those carrying out the mission of the Sisters of Providence, yesterday and today.

"I wonder if this is a "good sign" for being here?" I said to myself as we continued down the hallway. *"Could this be the answer to my prayer?"*

Dr Joseph Parazoo

There were four nurses around Kim when we entered the room. They were reciting "spelling bee" words and writing in their little pads. One male nurse had unwrapped her wrists. Then he started to draw an outline of the red areas. He told me that it was a way to see if the redness or infection was spreading.

They all continued to watch the monitors and writing in their pads. Once in a while they would ask us questions about the situation. After a few moments, they were all gone. *"Who wrote all over me?"* Kim said to herself when she looked at her wrists. *"I'm going to get in trouble for this."* She fell back into a deep sleep.

Dr. Good Hands was a fairly tall man in his late forties. It was about two o'clock in the afternoon. He was thin, clean shaved, and very confident. He was a skilled surgeon. This is the guy that is supposed to be the "best in the state." There was that "smell" of success about him. He also had the air of arrogance. I recognized that air right off; I suffer from the same ailment.

Dr. Disease Buster was an infectious disease specialist. He was also a tall, thin man. Clean shaved, and in his sixties. He was well dressed, yet the suit was outdated. With his slightly drooping shoulders, I pictured him spending a lot of time at his desk. He was one of those that would continuously be reading the *American Medical Journal*.

They were "consulting" with James and me, for it seemed like hours. It felt more like being in a courtroom, on the stand. I know that they were just trying to get a handle on the situation before they went into surgery. They explained that they would have to study the "case" and "examine" her. Then they would be able to answer some of our questions, and

Surviving MRSA

hopefully put a stop to this.

They were very concerned with the blood sugar thing. They seemed very surprised when I told them she was not a diabetic. They were planning to go into surgery at six o'clock.

"How long will the surgery be?"

"I won't know until I get a look at her. I would say, at least four hours. At this moment, all I have to work from is the reports. We are still waiting for test results," Dr. Good Hands responded. *"Do you have any more questions?"* .

"I can't think of any. Doc, do me a favor, bring her back to me."

"I won't promise anything, except I'll do my best. If there is nothing else, I'll talk to you when I get finished."

I just sat there for a few moments, thinking. The way he talked and carried himself, he must have been born with surgical experience. A tyrant in his operating room, a tiger, arrogant and a difficult man to work for. Yet, a top-notch surgical technician.

Someone I want, working on Kim... someone I want on my side. We all left the conference room. The two doctors off to study the case. Us two, off to worry and pace the floors.

The room was small, and seemed crowded. One bed in the middle, surrounded by machines. There was one nurse for each room, seated just outside. At least she looked like she was getting a peaceful rest, just lying there. The scene was different from this side, though. The situation appeared more serious here. She was still swelled up with excess liquid being pumped into her. *"Hi, honey,"* I said as I bent down and kissed her on the forehead.

There was a noisy machine in the corner. There was a tube the size of your thumb down her throat. Looking at the machine, it was forcing air into her lungs. *Why is it taped to*

Dr Joseph Parazoo

her mouth?
   She had a small tube snaked through her nose. It was filled with a nasty grayish-brown liquid. Following the tube, I saw that it is a feeding tube. *I guess they plan on having her asleep awhile.*
   There was a blood pressure cuff on her arm, leading to the monitor. The monitor beeped and flashed as it displayed the various readings of the heart rate, blood pressure, oxygen, etc. *That machine even has her temperature on it... One hundred two.*
   Look at all of those bags... I wonder what they contain? This one says, chemoprophylaxis. That one says insulin. This one here says glucose. This one over here says cephalosporin.
   There is another rack, This one says saline solution. That one says metronidazole. This one over here says immunoglobuin. Man, that's a lot of stuff.
   Hey, this room has a view. Why would a room in the intensive care need a window?
   I walked a little closer and took a look. *Six stories up, and view of the freeway. Nice.. Look at all of those computers, on the nursing station out there..... I wonder what is in this cabinet? Think I should look? Na, maybe later...... Man, I sure look tired...look at those dark circles under my eyes. Why is there a mirror in here, anyway? There's a chair...maybe I should sit down.* I reached for Kim's hand as I slid the chair closer.
   The nurses escorted everyone out of Kim's room at about 5:30; they had to prep her for the surgery. We decided to move the conversation down to the cafeteria for a while. Of course, once dinner was over, we moved back up to the waiting room.

Surviving MRSA

Dr Joseph Parazoo

Chapter Eight
The Symptoms

This is a portion from the National Necrotizing Fasciitis Foundation: Unfortunately necrotizing fasciitis often has flu-like symptoms, so initially, the natural assumption is for the individual to believe they have the flu. Often, NF occurs in otherwise healthy, active individuals. **No major trauma is necessary.**

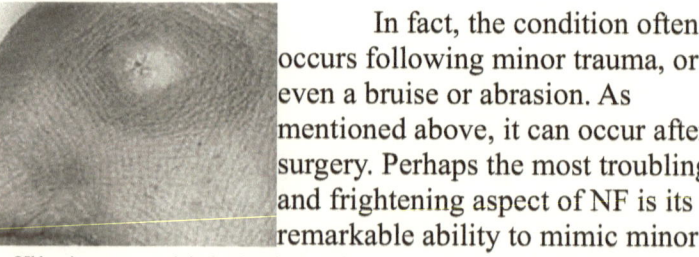

In fact, the condition often occurs following minor trauma, or even a bruise or abrasion. As mentioned above, it can occur after surgery. Perhaps the most troubling and frightening aspect of NF is its remarkable ability to mimic minor afflictions—which fools both the patient and the doctor.

Mis-diagnosis is very common, which, in light of the speed and deadliness of the infection, often has severe consequences, such as multiple limb amputation and too often, death. In post-surgical patients, NF often mimics common post-operative symptoms such as severe pain, inflammation, fever and nausea, which also thwarts a timely diagnosis.

Education and awareness by the general public as well as the medical community in recognizing symptoms is critical to saving lives.

Surviving MRSA

The following depicts general symptoms of NF as the disease advances.

Trauma (day zero). This "trauma" does not have to be major, like getting hit with a baseball bat, or a car accident; it could be as small as a bee sting, hemorrhoids, pimple, or ingrown hair.

Discomfort in the general region of the trauma (day zero).Pain that is out of proportion with the injury. Influenza-like symptoms such as vomiting, diarrhea, dehydration, malaise, weakness, muscle pain, and fever. Swelling or sunburn-type redness in the general region of the injured area (day two).

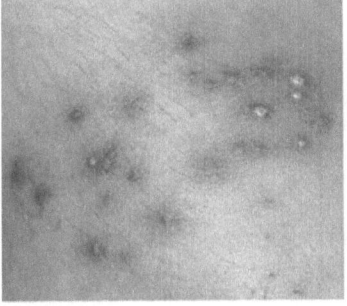

Dr Joseph Parazoo

Worsening of the condition. Less frequent urination. Large, boil-like blister(s) containing foul-smelling pus (day two to day three).

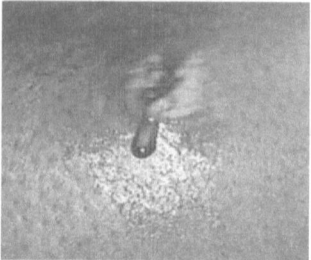

Hemorrhage or bursting of the blister. Gangrene (day four). Early signs and symptoms of streptococcal toxic shock syndrome (STSS): Fever. Dizziness. Confusion. A flat red rash over large areas of the body.

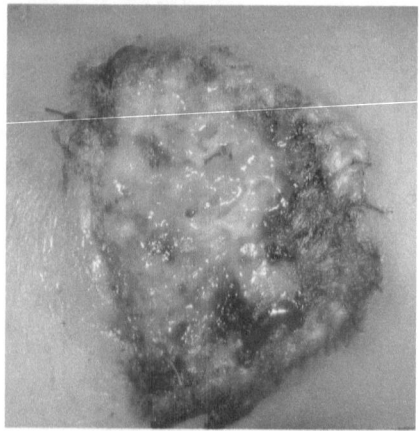

Surviving MRSA

Dr Joseph Parazoo

Chapter Nine
How It Spreads

Basically speaking, strep in any form is easy to spread. It is a very common bacteria that lives in and on people.

So, in order to keep from the bacteria developing into something more serious, you have to take care of your wounds. You have to maintain a daily cleansing routine. You should eat a "healthy" diet, in order to keep your immune system in top condition.

The strep bacteria is spread through direct contact, and occasionally through coughing, kissing and other mucous swapping activities. You can be a carrier of strep without showing any symptoms.

This common "bug," called strep, that causes strep throat, is a nasty bug. There are **over eighty types of this bacteria that are not affected by antibiotics**.

These bacteria cause problems that range from minor to very major problems. The scary thing is that it lives in and on us people, all the time. Just think, there are over 10 million minor cases of this "bug," just waiting for the "right circumstances" to develop into a major case.

It usually enters the human body where there is a break in the skin caused by injury. This includes cuts, burns, penetrating injuries, operative sites, enterostomy, blunt trauma, ulcers and diabetic feet. Once in the bloodstream, the bacteria moves rapidly through tissue in a path along the fascia, which is the subcutaneous tissue (just beneath the skin)

Surviving MRSA

surrounding the muscle. Rapid multiplication of this invading army causes antibodies to recognize them and to release chemicals that signal white blood cells to swallow the bacteria.

The following information was taken from the CDC:

These bacteria are spread through direct contact with mucus from the nose or throat of persons who are infected or through contact with infected wounds or sores on the skin. Ill persons, such as those who have strep throat or skin infections, are most likely to spread the infection.

In order for someone to contract NF, the bacteria must be introduced into the body. This occurs either from direct contact with someone carrying the bacteria, or because of the bacteria is being carried by the person him or herself.

The bacteria that produce the toxins that cause necrotizing fasciitis can be passed from person to person. However, a person who acquires the bacteria is unlikely to develop a severe infection unless he or she has an open wound, chicken pox, or an impaired immune system.

If you have direct close contact with someone that has necrotizing fasciitis, in the active stages, your doctor may want you to take antibiotics, as a precaution.

According to Dr. Dennis Stevens: History is replete with descriptions of epidemics of Group A Strep infections and their non-suppurative sequelae.

In the 1600s, epidemics of scarlet fever spread from Italy and Spain to Northern Europe, and in 1736, an outbreak occurred in the American colonies, killing 4,000 people.

Dr Joseph Parazoo

Major epidemics of rheumatic fever occurred in World War II in the U.S. military.

Soon afterward post-streptococcal glomerulonephritis struck several regions of the United States. More than 80 different M types of S. pyogenes exist. The complications of current Group A Strep infections are severe; bacteremia associated with aggressive soft tissue infection, shock, adult respiratory distress syndrome and renal failure are common; **30% to 70% of patients die** in spite of aggressive modern treatments.

Surviving MRSA

Dr Joseph Parazoo

Chapter Ten
Skills at Work

The double doors of the OR opened with a bang as the bed was pushed through. Meanwhile, dressed in the usual green scrub suit, Dr. Good Hands walked toward the scrub sink. His backup surgeon was beside him, performing the surgical scrub. *"I'm not sure what we are going to find. This is that transfer from Willamette Valley Medical Center."*

"Necrotizing fasciitis is never pretty." His scrub finished. Dr. Good Hands backed through the swinging doors into the operating room. He said good evening to the nurses and the anesthetist. Stopping briefly to put on his surgical gown and gloves. With ordinary operating room etiquette, the assistant had already draped the incision area.

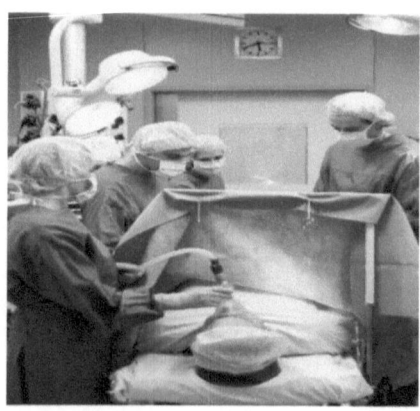

Surviving MRSA

"Scalpel," he said as he placed his palm upward. The scalpel was immediately placed in his hand. The scrub nurse had worked with Dr. Good Hands for many years. She always studied the particulars of the operation beforehand. She always knew what tools he would need, sometimes before he did.

With scalpel in hand, he made a four-inch incision in her abdomen.

"Retract." The scrub nurse took hold of the stainless-steel retractors and gently tugged the wound open.

"Scalpel." With her intestines in his hand, he made the proper incision.

"Suture." He poked the curved suture needle through the edge of the colon, and drew the thread tight. This was a simple colostomy. Dr. Good Hands snipped the needle and tied the last stitch.

"Re-drape," he commanded, and stepped away from the table. He doffed his gloves, and put on a fresh pair.

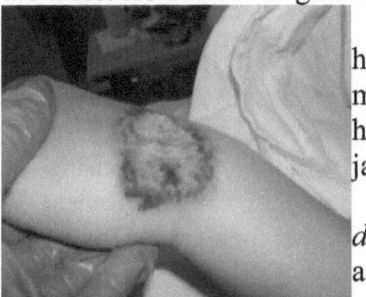

"Scalpel," he said as he approached the patient one more time. With the scalpel in hand, he carefully cleaned off the jagged edges of the wound.

"What were they thinking? I don't see any bacteria here," the assistant remarked.

"We can save the hand then." After he had cleaned up the wrist area, he barked, *"Re-drape."*

Dr. Good Hands stepped away from the operating table. He removed his gloves and put on a clean pair. While

Dr Joseph Parazoo

the assistant marked and draped the patient, another nurse bandaged the wrist.

Debridement is a term used by surgeons for the removing of grossly contaminated soft tissue. They remove the dead tissue to reveal a healthy bleeding wound surface. Surgical debridement is rapid and can involve the removal of large volumes of tissue at one time. Sharp debridement should be considered as the gold standard, as it can reduce the risk of wound complications and aid the healing process.

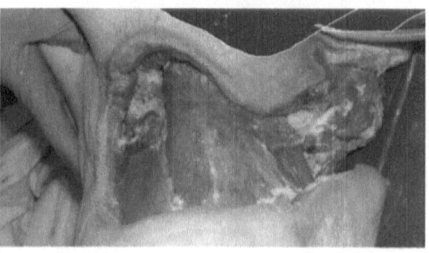

"Scalpel," he said as he stepped back to the table. With scalpel in hand, he took a delicate slice of the grayish, dead tissue. He had been using his surgical skills for over twenty years. He knew the anatomy of the human body very well. He didn't want to take any muscle if he didn't have to. He knew exactly how deep to make the cut.

Sharp debridement can produce rapid results. It requires a high level of skill and experience. Practitioners must have the necessary knowledge and training to complete the task safely and effectively. They should also be able to deal with the many possible complications as they arise.

"Suction," he commanded The scrub nurse was ready, and guided the suction tube over the open wound. The machine gurgled as the rusty blood and pieces of dead flesh traveled through the plastic hose.

"Reposition," he barked. He handed the scalpel back

Surviving MRSA

to the scrub nurse and stepped away from the table.

The scrub nurse glanced up and noticed the sweet drops forming on his forehead. Using a sterile cloth, she wiped it dry.

He had completed the procedure on the front side. He was waiting for the team to reposition her, so he could start on the worst part. He glanced up at the clock; two hours had passed. A slight smile crossed his face; he was working at record speed. The smile soon disappeared as he thought about the sepsis and what he might find.

Dead tissue acts as a medium for bacterial growth. He was working with excessive inflammatory response, which is a result from the presence of necrotic material, that adds to the systemic release of cytokines, such as tumor necrosis factor, and interleukins which promote the septic response.

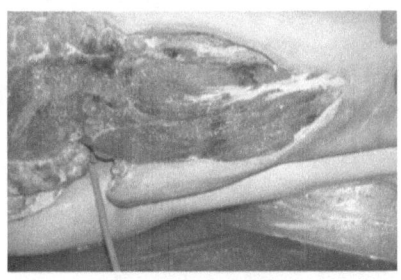

"Scalpel," he called as he approached the operating table. With scalpel in hand, he made a bold cut along the edge of the soft tissue.

He removed a large section of the grayish-black dead tissue. He could see that the bacteria had already made their way further along the skin.

One problem with this type of disease is time. The bacteria form bonds with each other. They systematically attach themselves to the healthy tissue. They smother this tissue to death, by starving it of vital oxygen.

"Suction," he commanded as he removed his hands

Dr Joseph Parazoo

from the wound area.

    In these cases, the surgeon is like a general in the army. The bacteria, the dreaded enemy. They are stealthy, and hide under the skin. They are quick, and spread rapidly. They can travel along the paths of the subcutaneous tissue, and attack in another area.
    They leave behind, in their wake, a deadly byproduct. This byproduct causes disturbances in other parts of the body. Time is their friend; the more time they have, the more casualties they have.
    The surgeon has one weapon, the scalpel. He has to rely mostly on his knowledge and his skill. The surgeon has to think and act fast. He has to find and cut the enemy off. He has to get behind the enemy lines, and destroy their home base.

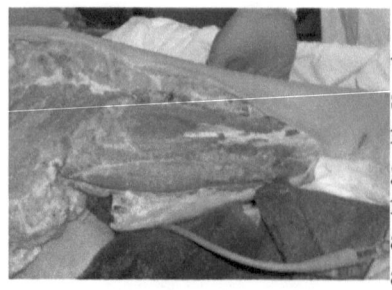

    The scrub nurse dabs the sweat from his brow with a sterile cloth. He makes another radical slice, eliminating the gray flesh, to expose the fresh meat of the muscle. He will try and save as much of the tissue as he can. Yet, wanting to eradicate the enemy, he will take everything that he has to.

    Beep… Beep… "She's losing pressure."
    "Turn that IV up… Get some more fluids into her."
    Dr. Good Hands takes a deep breath, and continues his search. The scalpel makes another sweep along the edge the her leg. He separated the gray tissue, from the pink flesh.
    "Suction," he said as he withdrew his hands. The

Surviving MRSA

scrub nurse was ready with the suction tube, and started to remove the excess blood from the gaping wound.

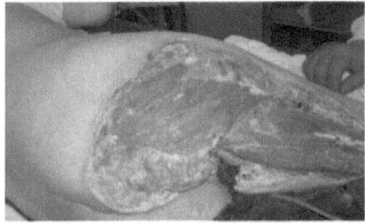

Dr. Good Hands stepped up to the operating table and resumed. A slice here, and swipe there, there was more than he anticipated. *That surgeon wasn't aggressive enough.*

Another day, he would have lost her, he thought to himself as he cut another section of the tissue. He continued to work fast, yet with great care.

The final cut was made. Dr. Good Hands left the operating room, stripping off his gloves and gown as he went. He proceeded to the locker room for a cup of coffee. The assistant would finish cleaning the area. Then the nurses could bandage her up.

It was about 11:30, when Dr Good Hands came out to the waiting room. That was about five and a half hours worth of surgery.

"*For the most part, I would say that it was a successful operation. The first thing I did, was to insert a colostomy bag. That will keep the area cleaner. I don't know what they were thinking on the wrist. I couldn't find any bacteria there. I moved the IV from her chest and placed it in her neck. That can come out in a few days."*

"*What about the spot on her butt?"*

"*I preformed debridement on the site. I removed more of the superficial fascia. Luckily we didn't have to touch any*

Dr Joseph Parazoo

muscle. I preformed debridement on the leg area, as well. Most of my time was spent cleaning up the areas, and searching for hidden bacteria. I had to go further down her leg."

"How far down?"

"About three quarters of the way to her knee."

"You said that she isn't stable yet. What does that mean?"

"Her blood pressure is low. We can't regulate her glucose levels yet. She is totally dependent on the ventilator. There may be some bacteria, still hiding."

"So, does that mean that there could be more surgery?"

"Very possible. We aren't completely out of the woods. We might have to do another debridement. It's one of those wait and see things."

"Is she going to be all right?"

"At this point, I couldn't say. I'm doing my best to save her life. She is a tough gal. But, at this point...I don't know if I can even save her leg. This is a wait-and-see thing. This necrotizing fasciitis stuff moves very fast. In the meantime, we are doing everything that we can."

"And what would that be?"

"A broad spectrum of antibiotics, radical debridement, or possible amputation... we may try using the hyperbolic chamber... but for now, there are too many machines that she is depending on.... we will do whatever may be necessary to save her life. Are there any questions?" Not finding any, Dr. Good Hands left the room.

We took our turns visiting with Kim and discussed the new information that we were faced with. It was still hard to believe that just a few days ago she was fine. Now, with all of the technology, she was near death.

Surviving MRSA

Dr Joseph Parazoo

Chapter Eleven
Strep A

According to the CDC: Group A streptococcus (GAS) is a bacterium often found in the throat and on the skin. People may carry group A streptococci in the throat or on the skin and have no symptoms of illness. Most GAS infections are relatively mild illnesses such as "strep throat," or impetigo. On rare occasions, these bacteria can cause other severe and even life-threatening diseases.

Staph infections hit 12 Million every year

With the dog days of summer and warm-weather sports in full swing, it's important to pay special attention to cuts, bruises and rashes that occur along with the fun. Staph — one of the most common skin infections in the United States — is responsible for 12 million to 14 million doctors' visits each year.

Close contact with others, sports that involve skin-to-skin contact, and warm, humid environments are a fertile breeding ground for staph infections. Staph bacteria can live harmlessly on many skin surfaces, especially around the nose, mouth, genitals and anus.

Listen to what the British Broadcasting Corporation has to say: Normally a harmless inhabitant of the mouth and upper respiratory tract, rogue S pyogenes is immensely destructive. It causes, among other things, strep throat (streptococcal pharyngitis), acne, rheumatic fever, toxic shock syndrome and—most horrifyingly—necrotizing fasciitis.

Surviving MRSA

It usually enters the human body where there is a break in the skin caused by injury. This includes cuts, burns, penetrating injuries, blunt trauma, operative sites, enterostomy, ulcers and diabetic feet. Once in the bloodstream, the bacteria moves rapidly through tissue in a path along the fascia, which is the subcutaneous tissue (just beneath the skin) surrounding the muscle. Rapid multiplication of this invading army causes antibodies to recognize them and to release chemicals that signal white blood cells to swallow the bacteria.
    In the case of S pyogenes infection, they pose a "digestive problem." An important cell wall component is very resistant to digestion, and will persist for as long as 146 days! These cells are leaky, and enzymes that leak out from it will cause, among other things, local damage to collagen fibres and the connective tissue matrix. However, all pathogenic strains of S pyogenes have a protein called M protein, which enables them to escape from being eaten.
    For more information on this "M Protein," look at the upcoming section entitled "MRSA." That section will definitely open your eyes.

    According to the National Institutes of Health: Group A streptococcal (strep) infections are caused by group A streptococcus, a bacterium responsible for a variety of health problems.
    These infections can range from a mild skin infection or sore throat to severe, life-threatening conditions such as toxic shock syndrome and necrotizing fasciitis, commonly known as flesh eating disease. Most people are familiar with strep throat, which along with minor skin infection, is the most common form of the disease. Health experts estimate that more than 10 million mild infections (throat and skin)

Dr Joseph Parazoo

like these occur every year.

According to Dr. Dennis Stevens: History is replete with descriptions of epidemics of Group A Strep infections and their non-suppurative sequelae. In the 1600s, epidemics of scarlet fever spread from Italy and Spain to Northern Europe, and in 1736, an outbreak occurred in the American colonies, killing 4,000 people. Major epidemics of rheumatic fever occurred in World War II in the U.S. military.
Soon afterward post-streptococcal glomerulonephritis struck several regions of the United States. More than 80 different M types of S. pyogenes exist. The complications of current Group A Strep infections are severe; bacteremia associated with aggressive soft tissue infection, shock, adult respiratory distress syndrome and renal failure are common; 30% to 70% of patients die in spite of aggressive modern treatments.

I have heard of those "old" diseases, and thought that they were eradicated. Apparently I was wrong; they are still alive, kicking ass and taking names. And did you see that line? There are more than 80 different M types of this bacteria that exist.

The Baylor College of Medicine in Houston, Texas, has done some molecular research and has this to say:
Serotype M1 group A Streptococcus, the most common cause of invasive disease in many case series, generally have resisted extensive molecular sub-typing by standard techniques. Statistics gathered by the Texas Department of Health indicated that from December 1, 1997, through March 5, 1998, 117 invasive episodes of GAS (and 26 deaths) had occurred statewide.

Surviving MRSA

Dr Joseph Parazoo

Chapter Twelve
Squabbles

It was about 3:00 before I finally crawled into bed. I hadn't really slept much in the past three days. I was completely exhausted. *"With the family here, I should sleep good."*
I was wrong; the body was running on overtime, completely on adrenalin. My mind would not shut off; the thoughts kept rolling in. Finally about 4:00, I dozed off.

It is pitch-black, only a shimmer of light from the stars. I find myself looking for something. It is terribly important to find, but I don't know what it is. I find myself looking in empty rooms, and through doors that lead nowhere. Occasionally, I glimpse something in the shadows. A frantic yet hopeless search for that which I have lost. At 6:00 in the morning I awoke, grunting and tussling briefly with the tangled sheets.

For the most part, it was an uneventful day. The family was still around, and that helped in passing the time away. There was a time that several of us were in visiting with Kim. Kathy and James were having some kind of a problem, and were arguing. I heard.

"Mom won't be able to work anymore," Kathy said.
"Maybe she will," James replied.
"She probably won't even be able to walk," Kathy retaliated.
"Don't say that. You don't know."
When I heard that, coupled with the other negative

Surviving MRSA

comments in the last couple of days, I took everyone out of the room. I made the following statements, rather harshly:
"If you guys want to fight, do it somewhere else. I do not want to hear negative talk of any kind, while you are in with your mother. She can hear everything that we say. She doesn't need to hear that negative stuff. When you are talking in that room you will talk positive, as if everything is all right!.

"But, it's true...she might not walk," Kathy responded.

"So? She doesn't need to hear that. Your job, while you are visiting her, is to show your love and to support her. To get her through this. She needs to hear only positive things. **Is that clear?** *"*

I didn't even wait for a response, I walked out of the ICU. I decided to go get a cup of coffee, and "cool off." The nursing staff must have overheard my conversation. Most of the negative talk around Kim stopped.

The doctors informed me that they ran further tests. I wondered if it had anything to do with some of the comments and questions that were made.

"Kim is what we call insulin resistant. Her pancreas still works, and produces some insulin. The problem is, she doesn't make enough."

"So, this diabetic thing...is temporary?"

"Probably not; she is a type II diabetic."

"While I have you here, what is that IV bag labeled Fentanyl for?"

"That is a heavy-duty pain medication, similar to Demerol." I found out later, that *Fentanyl* is 10 times more potent than *Morphine* and 100 times as addictive.

One of the nurses brought in some boots to help keep

Dr Joseph Parazoo

the circulation going in Kim's feet. We were told that the longer a person did not have any movement, the more atrophy would set in. Atrophy is the wasting away of muscles that are not used.

What happens is the body notices that these muscles are not needed. So, it starts a degeneration process, it takes the "building blocks" from the muscles, and uses them somewhere else.

These boots were real pretty, and blue. They had a hard sole, an open toe, and the rest was made of a canvas-type material. There was a flat metal rod on either side to help keep the foot straight with the leg. Once the boots were in place, the Velcro flaps held them in place. There was a small air tube attached. The air pressure cycled through, releasing and re-inflating the boots. The main purpose of these is to keep the circulation going.

"How long is she gong to be in here?"
"She's going to be here a long time."

Not knowing how long Kim would be in this situation, we started to take turns at massaging her feet. We also started to exercise her legs.

By the end of the day, the doctors had decided that she was improving. That she was "out of the woods," so to speak…for now. Basically, that meant she could still need more surgery. But, she was no longer in grave danger of death. They were still having problems regulating the blood sugar. Her blood pressure was more stable.

Surviving MRSA

Dr Joseph Parazoo

Chapter Thirteen
Strep B

According to DHPE: Strep B streptococcus, or group B strep, is a bacterium that causes life-threatening infections.

Many people carry the group B strep bacteria in their bodies, without developing infections or illness. However, the bacteria can become deadly, to people with weakened immune systems. Group B strep is the most common cause of sepsis (infection of the blood), among newborns. Group B strep is also a common cause of pneumonia.

Group B strep bacteria are different from many other types of bacteria. People can be "colonized" with the group B strep. This means that they carry the bacteria in their bodies. But, are not infected and do not become sick. Adults can carry the bacteria in the gastrointestinal tract, genital tract, or the urinary tract. About 10% to 30% of the pregnant women are colonized with group B strep, in the genital tract.

Colonization with group B strep is usually harmless. The bacteria can become deadly, though, if something happens that allows them to invade the bloodstream. Most adults usually show no signs or symptoms. however, in rare infections, urinary tract infections, skin infections, and pneumonia. Group B strep infection is fatal in about 20% of infected men, and non-pregnant women.

Since 1970, disease from group B strep, has been on the rise. Starting with only 18,000 cases in the United States. The number of adult cases, was doubled by 1980.

Surviving MRSA

Dr Joseph Parazoo

Chapter Fourteen
Progress

While changing her bandages, the doctors noticed that there was some more dead tissue. They scheduled another debridement surgery for the afternoon.

Monday didn't seem that much busier than the weekend. It was somewhere after 11:00, when the blood pressure section started to flash and beep. The number was rapidly changing, of a range between thirty-eight and forty-six. The nurses didn't talk about it as if it was a problem. However, I did notice that they spent more time watching and checking the monitor.

They informed us about the upcoming surgery. It was scheduled for 2:00. They said that the wound didn't look too bad, and they shouldn't be very long. They didn't want the bacteria to take hold again and get out of hand. The total wait time, from prep to Kim being back in her room, was only about an two hours.

"Are you ready to do this? One, two, three, and move." The four pairs of hands, in one smooth motion, slid the woman from the bed, unto the operating table.

His scrub finished, Dr. Good Hands backed through the swinging doors into the operating room. He said good afternoon to the nurses and the anesthetist. Stopping briefly to put on his surgical gown and gloves. With ordinary operating room etiquette, the assistant had already draped the incision area.

Surviving MRSA

"*Scalpel.*" The scalpel was immediately placed in his hand, by the scrub nurse. With scalpel in hand, he took a delicate slice of the grayish, dead tissue. With precision, he cleaned the edges of the wound, removing the dead flesh.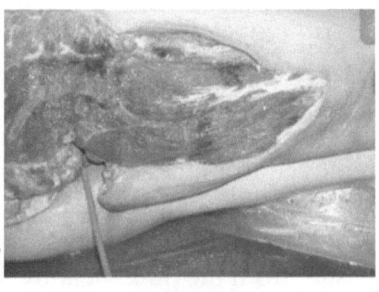
The scrub nurse swabbed the moisture from his forehead. He slowly surveyed the area, looking for the telltale sign of the bacteria. It didn't take long to locate the damage.
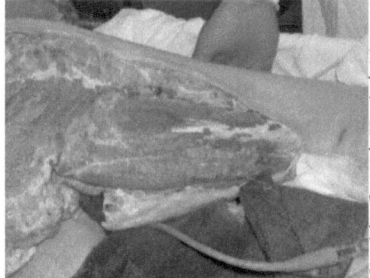 The bacteria had already made its way further down the leg. Nested just under the fold of the skin, was a large pocket of bacteria. He took another slice of the decaying flesh, removing more of the subcutaneous tissue, all the way down to the muscle.
"*Suction,*" he said as he withdrew his hands. The scrub nurse was ahead of him again. She placed the suction tube on the open wound. The machine gurgled as the blood traveled through the plastic tube. Once she removed the suction tube, the surgeon continued his work.
Beep.... "*She's losing pressure*"
"*Get those fluids in her. Turn that IV up.*"
Dr. Good Hands took another cut along the edge of the wound. He was getting close to the knee, the depth had to be precise. He thought to himself as he worked, *Have to be careful not to cut the tendons.... Steady.*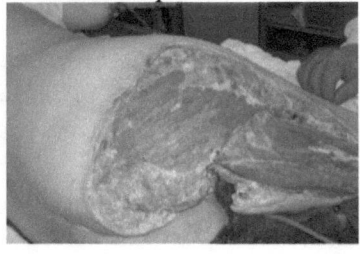

Dr Joseph Parazoo

... Not too deep.... Perfect. The scrub nurse took a sterile cloth and wiped the moisture from his forehead.

"Suction." The gurgle of the machine filled the room as the rusty blood, along with pieces of gray flesh, was removed from the open wound.

With scalpel in hand, he separated the gray, dead tissue, from the pink, healthy tissue.

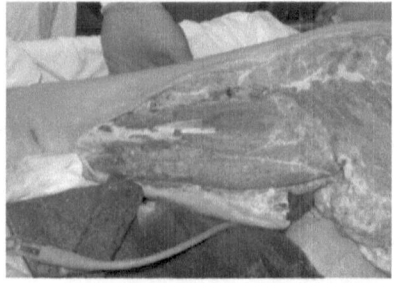

"Suction," he said as he backed away from the operating table. He slowly stripped off his rubber gloves, removed his bloodstained gown, cap, and his mask. He headed for the surgical locker room to change and get a cup of coffee. He knew that the nurses would take care of the bandaging.

Dr. Good Hands walked into the waiting room and greeted us.

"How is Kim doing?"

"She is getting better. She doesn't have as much septicemia as before. I had to remove a little more subcutaneous tissue from the back of her leg. I was able to stop just above her knee.

"I noticed that her blood pressure was pretty low today."

"Most of that was caused by the sepsis. I think we have that under control...now."

"Do you have any idea as to how long she will be here?"

"Not at this time. It will depend on what happens in the next couple of days."

Surviving MRSA

Kim slowly opened her eyes and looked around. Seeing those all-too-familiar tubes, lines, and... those machines. *Are all of those machines, for me? I must have had a heart attach. What else could it be?* She drifted back into the darkness. She had seen her father in similar situations many times over the years.

One of the hospital priests walked by the room. Sylvia stopped her, and asked if she could pray for Kim. The priest reached into a small bowl, and placed the sign of the cross on Sylvia's forehead.
"In the name of the Father, the Son, and the Holy Spirit." About that time, Kim felt the presence of something and opened her eyes.
"Can I have some, too?" Kim asked. Sylvia and the priest turned with startled looks on their faces.
"Sure," was the reply as the priest walked toward Kim.
"In the name of the Father, the Son, and the Holy Spirit," the priest said as she placed the sign of the cross on Kim's forehead. After a short prayer, the priest left to continue on her rounds. Meanwhile, Kim felt at peace and drifted back into her dreams.

The sun had gone down, and the lights were dimmed. The ICU was quieter than usual today. I sat comfortably in the recliner, all stretched out. The red lights flickered on the IVAC machine. The blinks of the rhythmic cycles were soothing, as it allowed the medicine to drip through the IV tubes.
They took the IV out of her neck. They put what they call a "pick line" in her upper arm. It operated like a permanent IV, only it was capped until they needed it. There

Dr Joseph Parazoo

were two connections attached to it. These connections were for plugging in the IV tubes. She still had to deal with the ventilator tube down her throat. The feeding tube still made its way through the nose. The number of bags had decreased to four.

The ventilator delivered its twenty breaths per minute. Each whoosh followed by the sigh, with the deflation of the ribs and the chest wall. It was easy to synchronize my breathing with the machine. The silvery moonlight, shimmered through the window.

The smell of fresh-baked bread, filled the room.
"Dinner will be ready in a minute." I glanced over, and Kathy was reading a book. James was playing with some truck. Victor was curled up in front of the stove.
"Did you need a hand, hon?" I asked as she scurried around the kitchen.
"You can cut the roast, if you want."

"Cough... Cough." The ventilator startled me, with the racket of the machine. It indicated that there was a problem. The nurse came in and cleaned Kim's airways so she could breathe again.

After the surgery on Monday, things started to improve. Every day, Kim seemed to get a little better. You could see that the swelling was coming down. Her skin was beginning to have that soft feel. Before, her skin was so tight that it almost felt like rubber. Her face started to get back some of that "rosy" look. The nurses had been kind of complaining that I would show up every day and spend a lot of time with Kim.

Kim slowly opened her eyes. She blinked several times, to adjust her focus. She lifted both of her arms about a

Surviving MRSA

foot off the bed. As she twisted and looks at her wrists, she thought, *What happened to my wrists? I know I didn't do that to myself. What the hell happened? I went into the hospital for a wound on my ass.* She drifted back to sleep as her hands dropped back to her side.

Kim slowly opened her eyes and looked around. *Where are they taking me?* She asked herself as she watched the ceiling moving past her. She heard several women talking, but couldn't really make out what they were saying. She drifted off into the darkness.

Once they reached the exam room, they took turns washing, and pulled on rubber gloves. As the nurses rolled Kim onto her side, she heard them talking.

"Why don't you change the catheter while we get this sheeting ready." She was still very disoriented, and wondered, *I know what a catheter is. What sheeting are they talking about?*

About that time, she heard what she thought was cellophane plastic being unrolled. Her senses faded out again into silence. The nurses continued their mission as the guest specialist explained the process. Upon completion, they removed their gloves, and started the travel back to the ICU room.

The sunlight peered through the window, and created a glare on the television. Kim opened her eyes and blinked. She immediately squinted from the glare. As she looked around the room, everything was fuzzy. *Where am I?* she asked herself. Everything had a kind of glow to it. She tried to fight the heaviness of her eyes. Her strength was low, but the darkness won over.

"Hello, hon," I said as I grabbed her hand. Without

Dr Joseph Parazoo

waking, she squeezed my hand a little. Her color was almost normal. I felt the smile of my face widen, there was a feeling…of something…of relief.

We found out that they decided to try a new machine on her. They called it a "wound-vac."

First, they take all of the bandages off. They place a thin black "sponge-like" sheet over the wound. This is then covered with a piece of plastic sheeting. A small hose is then attached to this plastic sheeting. The hose is connected to the machine. The machine works like a vacuum, and cycles through a suction process. This suction process pulls blood from the body, increasing the blood supply to the wound area.

This increases the healing process. At the same time, this machine pulls excess liquid, dead cells, etc. away from the wound. This keeps the wound dryer, less chance for infection to set in.

There is a "catch" bag that collects all of this liquid stuff. They empty and examine this "discharge" a couple of times a day.

The sun is shining brightly, a few small fluffy clouds are present in the sky. The soft breeze from the gulf whisks across the sand. I look over at James, as my dad is burying him. The sand must be very warm, as James starts to fall asleep. That looks so cute, I think I'll take a picture. Caption for the picture, *James and his grandpa, August 1982, Corpus Christi.* Kathy is running away from the surf, with a small bucket of water. As she approaches, she throws the water on her dad. Mom is sitting on a towel, reading a book. Everyone is enjoying this wonderful day on the beach.

Kim opened her eyes, blinked a couple of times to

Surviving MRSA

focus. Looking around, she thought, *This isn't Texas. This is a hospital. What am I doing here?*
"*Hello, hon. How are you doing?*"
"*Hold me,*" she said.
"*Sure,*" I replied as I leaned over the bed and put my arms around her.
"*Mmmmm. That's nice.*"
"*Yes, it is.*"
"*Just being held,*" she said as she continued to squeeze hard.
"*I'm here, hon...I'm not going anywhere.*"
"*I feel better already. Just knowing that you are here.*"
"*Everything is going to be all right.*"
"*As long as I have you.*"
"*Forever, and ever.*" I felt her grip release. Her arms fell back to the bed. Kim fells back into a deep sleep.

After some time, Kim lifted both of her arms about a foot off the bed. As she twisted and looked at her wrist, she thought, *What happened to my wrists? I went into the hospital for a wound on my ass. I know I didn't do that to myself. What the hell happened?* She drifted back to sleep.

Things were looking up. Most of the excess liquid was gone. She wasn't strong enough to eat on her own yet, so she still had to deal with the feeding tube. The breathing tube that was down her throat was removed. She was able to breathe on her own.

While we were all out to lunch, Kim looked around. She knew that she was in a hospital; she remembered going in. There was a "peel off" type calendar on the wall; it said

Dr Joseph Parazoo

seven. *What month? What year? How long have I been in here?* She thought to herself as she continued to survey the room.

The ICU was still and quiet; most of the lights were dim. It was about 1:00 in the morning. Kim was awakened by a familiar song. Across the hall, in one of the other rooms, were some people.
She blinked her eyes several times to get rid of the fuzziness. There were seven or eight people, dressed in black, crowded around the bed. *Someone must have died. Why else would they play taps over the speaker system? That is kind of strange. God, don't let them stop at my room!* Her vision started to fade out as she entered the blackness once more.
Somewhere around seven o'clock in the morning, a nurse with blond dreadlocks, walked into Kim's room. *"Good morning, sunshine. I brought you some orange juice. Do you remember where you are?"*
"A hospital. How long have I been here?" Kim responded,
"The first time I seen you was Thursday. Can you tell me what kind of juice this is? They are going to move you to your own room today."

According to the research, a metabolic disturbance can be induced by "sepsis." This sepsis is the toxic gases that are released from the bacteria that caused the infection. They continuously mention that organ failure can occur during the development of necrotizing fasciitis.

Surviving MRSA

Dr Joseph Parazoo

Chapter Fifteen
Crossed Wires

The doors of the ICU opened up to let us pass. We hung a left, and traveled past the waiting room and down the hall. After another left, we waited in front of an elevator. The elevator ride was short, and soon we entered a different wing. The halls were narrow, and patients were walking around.

The room was small, maybe twelve feet square. There was a bathroom on the left, just inside the door. There was a counter running the length of the bathroom wall. A couple of wooden cabinets decorated the east wall. There was a window that covered the north wall.

Running the length of the window was a bench-style cabinet. We found a few blankets, in case she was cool. Kim seemed to be in good spirits and wanted to talk. Her condition must be improving; she was no longer in the ICU. I felt a big sense of relief, and almost sighed.

We passed the rest of the afternoon in conversation. I noticed that once in a while, Kim would stop talking in the middle of a sentence. I didn't think much of it at the time. She appeared to be in that "thinking" mood, for a few moments, then she would continue.

Sometime after dinner, we are all crowded around Kim's bed, talking. Right in the middle of a sentence, she stopped talking. I saw that she started to raise her right arm. It was stiff and moving very slowly. She continued to raise it up, and then over her head.

She had this weird sort of shocked look of surprise on her face. She rolled her eyes to the right and looked at

Surviving MRSA

her arm. She didn't say anything; the look told me everything. Kim questioned herself, *What the hell is going on? I am not trying to move my arm.*

When the hand rested on the bed above her head, I noticed that all of the muscles in her legs were tense and quaking. She had a pale, frightened look on her face. She was having a seizure. I had dealt with seizure victims before, I knew what to do.

"She is having a seizure, We need to put something in her mouth. Zack, could you find something? Mom, hold her arm and leg still, if you can."

"*I'll bet it was the MS-Contin,*" Sylvia demanded.

According to Nemours Foundation: Seizures are caused by abnormal electrical discharges in the brain. Symptoms may vary depending on the part of the brain that is involved, but seizures often cause unusual sensations, uncontrollable muscle spasms, and loss of consciousness. Some seizures may be the result of a medical problem.

Low blood sugar, infection, a head injury, chemical imbalance in the blood, accidental poisoning, or drug overdose can cause a seizure. In addition, anything that results in a sudden lack of oxygen to the brain can cause a seizure. In some cases, the cause of the seizure is never discovered.

This was a mild, seemingly controlled seizure. It wasn't that wild and thrashing type that most people have. After we got her calmed down, I went to get the nurse.

After explaining what went on, the nurse didn't believe that she had a seizure, because she was still awake.

"*Has she had seizures before?*"

"*No...this is the first time.*"

"*I'll stay in here for a few minutes...to see if it*

Dr Joseph Parazoo

happens again."
   "*Shouldn't you be calling a doctor or something?"*
   "*The doctors are done for the day. She will be okay."*
   "*No, you will go get someone! Now!"* The nurse stomped out of the room.
   A few moments later, the floor supervisor came by and he watched Kim for a few moments. *"I don't see anything wrong. If you want, we can run some tests tomorrow."*
   I took him aside and proceeded to talk at him. I tried to keep my cool, and stay polite. *"I don't care what you have to do, or who you have to call. There is something wrong here...and I want you to run some tests, and find out what is going on.... Now!"*
   A few minutes later, two nurses started to push Kim's bed back toward the ICU. The doors of the elevator closed behind them. Kim started to scream in a low tune. She noticed that she was having another seizure.
   "*You are okay.... We are here."*
   "*What is going on?"* she asked, rather frightened.
   Within a few minutes, she was back in the intensive care unit. The doctor "in charge" was watching and examining Kim. She tried to explain that she couldn't have had a seizure if she was awake.
   While she was explaining this to me, Kim had another seizure, while being wide-awake. The doctor gave her some medication and started to set up a few tests. With all of things going on, the evening shortly turned into morning.
   I am not sure how many or what kind of tests that they ran. All I know is that every time that they would get the results of a test, they would say something along the lines of,
   "I don't know what is causing this; the tests come out negative."
   "I need you to run a STAT CT head scan," I overheard

Surviving MRSA

a nurse on the phone. It wasn't too long before they were wheeling her bed off for another test.

The neurologist slowly inserted the needle between the third and fourth lumbar vertebrae. This is called a lumbar puncture, sometimes, a spinal. He slowly pulled the plunger, and withdrew some of the spinal fluid.

The normal cerebro-spinal fluid contains various chemicals, such as protein and sugar (glucose), and few if any cells. The spinal fluid also has a normal pressure when first removed.

Upon running various tests, everything appeared normal. They told us that they would continue to find out what was going on. They were going to take her for an MRI. The process takes a while, and the results would take some time. That we should go home and get some sleep.

There wasn't a lot of things that we could do. We weren't able to see Kim while they did these tests. So, we decided to go. We walked out of the hospital about 3:00 that morning. Since it was so early, we decided to stop for breakfast.

I walked back into the hospital about 7:30. When I walked into Kim's room, it looked like a tornado had hit. All of the machines were off. The blood pressure cuff was lying on the floor. My first thought was, *What the hell happened here…. How are they monitoring her progress?* In a different part of the room, there was a pillow and a sheet on the floor.

"Morning, hon," I said as I walked over to Kim and kissed her. I could tell that she was a little upset, just by the

expression on her face. She was lying real close to the edge of the bed, her arms were crossed, and she was holding on to the railing. Kim opened her eyes, blinked a couple of times to focus.

"*Hello, hon. How are you doing?*" I asked, when I saw that she was awake.

"*Hold me,*" she said.

"*Sure,*" I replied as I leaned over the bed and put my arms around her.

"*That feels nice.*"

"*Yes, it does.*"

"*Just being held,*" she said as she continued to squeeze hard.

"*I know what you mean.*"

"*I feel better already. Just knowing that you are here.*"

"*Everything is going to be all right.*"

"*As long as I have you.*"

"*Forever, and ever.*" I felt that her grip release.

"*Get me out of here... That nurse is a bitch.*" The tone of her voice changed.

"*I know you do want out, I can't right now. Have you ate yet?*" I asked.

"*No.*" Kim replied

"*I'll go see if we can get something. I'll be back in a second,*" I said as I walked out of the room. I located the nurse and asked what had happened. The nurse said that Kim was being a bitch and tried to get out of bed. She wasn't going to go back in there until shift change at 8:00.

"*Can I get something? She is hungry.*"

"*What do you want?*"

"*I don't care...yogurt, pudding, something easy.*" I walked back into the room, to spend some time with Kim.

Surviving MRSA

"That bitch tied me in bed."
"She said that you tried to get out of bed."
"I did not. I can't go anywhere...my legs won't work. I was cold, and asked for a blanket. She called me a big baby, and tied me up. I want out of here. I'm mad. You have to tell them that I'm not stupid. They keep saying that I had a stroke."
"Who's saying that you had a stroke?"
"All of the nurses. They think that I'm dumb. I didn't have a stroke...and I'm not stupid. You have to tell them."
"Okay, hon...Calm down, I'll tell them."

I went out and talked to the nurse. I wanted to talk to someone in charge. She said that she would get someone as soon as she could. Within a few minutes, the supervising doctor came over.

I was just about to open my mouth, when he said, *"I have good news. A bed has opened up in the burn center over at Emanuel Hospital. They are much better equipped to deal with these types of wounds. They deal with this stuff all the time. We will start to prep her for transport soon. I wish you a speedy recovery and all the best to your family."*

After all of that, I decided it wouldn't do much good to make waves. I walked back into Kim's room and informed her of the transfer. With all the things that had happened in the past couple of days, I was glad.

Maybe Emanuel would be better.

Dr Joseph Parazoo

Surviving MRSA

Dr Joseph Parazoo

Chapter Sixteen
Dreaming

Kim wasn't feeling quite "all there" when she opened her eyes. She looked around and surveyed the ambulance. She began to think to herself, *This must be a dream. It feels like I am in a sardine can. This can't be a real ambulance.. I have all this stuff on my chest and belly. They don't really do that. Do they?* She drifted back to sleep.

We were all set in the "new" room by lunchtime. Since Kim had the "wound-vac" on, they took her off of all the antibiotics. She still had to deal with the feeding tube. She was still receiving a continuous drip of insulin; her levels hadn't stabilized yet.

Not finding out what had caused the seizures, they put her on a anti-seizure pill. Most of her color was back, and most of the swelling had disappeared. We spent the afternoon getting used to the new room and nurses.

The lights were low, and the curtains were closed. All was quiet. Kim stirred and opened her eyes. She blinked a couple of times, trying to get the fuzz out. She slowly scanned the room with her eyes, not recognizing anything.

Where am I? It looks like a hospital room. But whose? As she twisted her neck toward the headboard, her eyes became heavy. She blinked a couple of times to fight the urge. When her face touched the pillow, she fell back asleep.

At about six o'clock in the evening, Dr. Graph walked in. He introduced himself as Kim's new doctor. He stood about five feet eight and was stocky. He kept his hair short,

Surviving MRSA

about a half an inch long. He was clean shaved, except for the neatly trimmed mustache and goatee.

Kim was still a little upset about all the things that had gone on in the past couple of days. She didn't want to talk to anyone that she didn't know. So, she rolled over on her side, facing away from the doctor, and refused to talk to him. She knew that if she looked at him, she would eventually talk.

I explained what had taken place at Providence. He said that he understood. But he didn't like the thought that she wouldn't talk to him.

"I will look into the seizure thing. I have gone over Kim's records. She has gone through a lot. Are there any questions that I can answer for you?"

"How long do you think that she will be in here?"

"I really won't know until I get a look at the wound. From what I've seen in the records, I could guess. After the wound has healed some, about two weeks, or so. She will probably have three or four more surgeries, consisting of skin grafts."

"Are these skin grafts really necessary?"

"No. The wound will heal on it own. But, having a skin graph will help it to heal faster. Plus, it won't look like a shark took a bite out of her."

"Makes sense. Whatever will get her healed faster is all right with me."

"These surgeries will be spaced a week or two apart, depending on how quick she heals. A couple of weeks after that, she will be moved to a rehabilitation center to recover. I would say that she will be out somewhere around the middle of June or July."

"How does skin grafting work?"

"We harvest a piece of skin from the donor site... either the leg or the back...in this case, probably the front of

Dr Joseph Parazoo

the same leg as her wound."
"How do you harvest the skin?"
"We use a machine, kind of like a potato peeler, and just slice a thin layer off of the area. Then we use another machine to poke holes in it and stretch it. We then glue, staple or sew the stretched skin onto the wounded area...and hope that it takes."
"What kind of success rate?"
"About half of the patients have thirty to fifty percent of the graft stick and take the first time. Another twenty-five percent of the people have fifty to seventy percent stick. Now only about ten percent of the people have over seventy percent stick. But, that is really good. There is no real way to tell how Kim's grafts will take."

It was a cold and blustery day; snow covered the ground. The crackle of the wood stove filled the air. The wind was whistling in the trees. If you listened hard enough, you could hear the leaves rustle as they blew across the icy snow. Out of the corner of her eye, she caught the glimpse of something. She turned her head toward the shadow.
    She could hardly make out the shape, as it was almost the same color as the snow. He immediately stopped, and their eyes met. They instantly made a connection, almost recognition. The door of the shed slammed shut. The moment was gone. She stood there, staring at the snow, searching, hoping that the fox would reappear. After a few moments, the wind picked up, and stirred the snow into a flurry.
    She found herself walking down a white-tiled hallway. Several bandaged people had risen up from the beds. She ran down the hallway, trying to get away. They started losing their bandages, exposing the gray tissue of dead flesh. She ran past the operating room. More people got up from the stainless-

Surviving MRSA

steel operating tables. They were searching for her; chunks of rotten flesh fell off of them as they followed.

The white tile glistened under the lightning strikes; it was the only time she could see. But, every time the light shone, she felt the current. It entered at her hip, went down through her leg, and out her knee. She continued to run through the hospital corridors, in an endless maze.

Wikipedia, the online encyclopedia, says that the following items can also cause seizures: Intoxication with drugs, drug toxicity, for example aminophylline or local anesthetics, normal doses of certain drugs that lower the seizure threshold, infection, metabolic disturbances, such as hypoglycemia or hypoxia, and the withdrawal from drugs.

Snap. The sudden noise woke Kim from her sleep. She tried to move, but she couldn't. *Why can't I move my legs, or my arms?* She lifted her head and took a survey. There was a leather strap on each leg, holding her to the bed. Looking at her arms, they were also strapped to the bed.

The room was dark, and quite, only a small creaking sound coming from her left side, up by her head. As she slowly twisted her neck to see, a human figure started to appear.

She was suddenly struck with the knowledge that there was danger. She experienced all of the involuntary animal reactions to the threat: a shiver up her spine; her scalp seemed to crawl and then tighten; her heart began to pound; her mouth went dry; her hands started to curl into claws; her hearing seemed to be more acute, and her eyes widened.

She saw a pair of hands holding a syringe. It was about an inch thick, and supported a large needle, and it was long. It was a woman, she had long, frizzy hair, and wore a

Dr Joseph Parazoo

devilish smile.

The woman took a step closer, and Kim noticed that she was wearing a green nurse's uniform. She watched as the needle was slowly lowered toward her arm. She started to squirm and thrash. But she couldn't get away. She let out a blood-curdling scream. Kim quickly opened her eyes, with a start, and tried to focus.

It was dark, only a small amount of the moonlight, shone through the window. The amber glow from the night-lights created shadows throughout the room. There was nobody in sight. She looked at her ankles and wrists...no restraints. *I need to get out of here.*

Her heart was still pounding. Her palms were damp and clammy as she grasped the handrails and pulled herself to the edge of the bed. She maneuvered her legs over the side and sat up. With both hands on the bed to steady herself, she started to move. Both of her feet touched the cool floor.

Why can't I feel the floor? Her legs were weak and felt like rubber as she tried to stand. The sheet was slippery and couldn't hold her. The booties that covered her feet didn't help. They were slippery against the waxed tile. She tried to steady herself, but she fell to her knees.

Just about that time, Jim, the nurse, walked in. *"Stay right where you are. I will get some help."* He reached over the bed, and pushed the call button. *"I need some help in room one."* Within moments, several nurses responded to the call. After they put Kim back into the bed, Jim made a nodding motion with his head.

"There is nothing to be afraid of," a calming male nurse voiced out. It briefly relaxed her, and stole her attention. Jim took a syringe out of his pocket. Pulling the cap off of the needle, he inserted it into the pick line. He slowly pushed the plunger. He put the syringe back in his pocket. He performed

Surviving MRSA

all this so quickly, that Kim didn't know about it.
"*Do you know where you are?*" Jim asked.
The room was dark, her vision was a blurry. She looked around, to get her bearings.
"*You're a medic, right?*"
"*Yes...of some sort.*"
"*I'm in Corpus Christi, at the airport.*"
"*What are you doing there?*"
"*Is something wrong with them?*"
"*Wrong with who?*"
"*Where are my babies? ...James, and Kathy!*"
"*I don't know James and Kathy.*" The sedative took effect, and did its job.... Kim drifted into the darkness.

Kim opened her eyes and blinked a couple of times to focus. Looking around, she thought, *This isn't Texas. This is a hospital. What am I doing here?*
"*Hello, hon. How are you doing?*" I asked.
"*Hold me,*" she said.
"*Sure,*" I replied as I leaned over the bed and put my arms around her.
"*That feels nice.*"
"*Yes. It does feel good..*"
"*Just being held,*" she said as she continued to squeeze hard.
"*I'm here.*"
"*I feel better already. Just knowing that you are here.*"
"*Everything is going to be all right.*"
"*As long as I have you.*"
"*Forever, and ever.*" I felt that her grip release. Her arms fell back to the bed. Kim fell back into a deep sleep.
About one o'clock in the afternoon, Dr. Graph walked

Dr Joseph Parazoo

in. He reported that, according to the reports, the seizures were probably caused by one of the antibiotics. With all of the tests that they ran, they weren't able to find any particular reason for the seizures.

> The Neurology Channel has this to say: Seizures can also occur in the normal nervous system when its metabolic balance is disturbed. The cause (etiology) of epilepsy may be not clearly known (idiopathic) or related to a particular disease state. About 35% of all cases of epilepsy have no clearly definable cause.
> Disorders that change levels of various metabolic substances in the body sometimes result in seizures; Altered levels of sodium, calcium, or magnesium (electrolyte imbalance), low blood sugar (hypoglycemia), or elevated blood sugar (hyperglycemia); Lowered oxygen level in the brain (hypoxia), and elevation of associated toxins. Overdose of and/or abrupt withdrawal from some prescription drugs can result in seizure activity.

Kim did not want to take the anti-seizure medication. The doctor agreed that it wasn't necessary, so they started to "wean" her off of them. We discussed the happening in the middle of the night.

"*Could Ms-Contin be cause hallucinations?*" I asked.
"*Very possible, it is a morphine derivative.*"
"*If the pain medicine is going to do that to me, I don't want any,*" Kim commented.
"*Okay, we can take you off of Ms-Contin. I'll leave a note with the nurses to use Oxycotin instead.*"
"*Can I refuse it?*" Kim asked.
"*You are the one to say how much pain you are in. If you don't think you need any…you don't have to take it.*"

Surviving MRSA

Dr Joseph Parazoo

Chapter Seventeen
Necrotizing Fasciitis

Necrotizing fasciitis (NECK-ro-tie-zing fash-ee-EYE-tiss) is the dreaded "flesh-eating virus" of supermarket tabloid fame. Unfortunately, while it really isn't a virus, but a bacterial infection, the fear is justified. While rare, this syndrome is devastating, disfiguring, and potentially lethal.

This is what British Broadcast Corporation has to say: Necrotizing fasciitis, caused by Streptococcus pyogenes, the flesh-eating bacteria, begins with a minor injury, usually on an extremity. Wounds of any sort will hurt, but in this case the pain is excruciating.

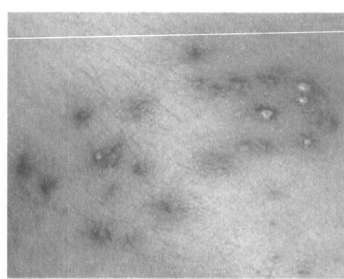

Fever begins to set in, and an unusual redness develops around the area of injury and rapidly moves away from the initial site.

By the next day, the redness has turned a strange blue color, and the skin begins to blister horribly, the bullae (blister) containing sickly yellowish to bluish fluid.

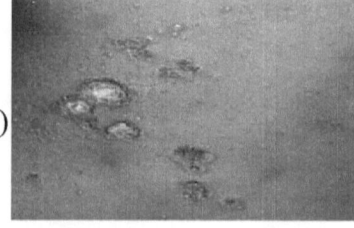

Surviving MRSA

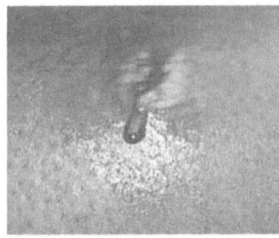

Some of these blisters may hemorrhage, causing an eruption of foul smelling pus and loss of copious amounts of blood. The pain at this point is severe, almost intolerable.

By day four, it is obvious that gangrene has set in, and massive sloughing of the skin occurs. At the hospital, surgeons plunge into a desperate, exhausting battle against the disease, fervently hacking away flesh that becomes rotten almost as fast as scalpels can cut it away. The prognosis is very poor, and the struggle for life continues until death or disfigurement comes— or maybe both.

According to Michael Maynor, MD, Clinical Assistant Professor, Department of Hyperbaric/Emergency Medicine, Louisiana State University School of Medicine: Necrotizing fasciitis is a progressive, rapidly spreading, inflammatory infection located in the deep fascia, with secondary necrosis of the subcutaneous tissues. Because of the presence of gas-forming organisms, subcutaneous air is classically described in necrotizing fasciitis.

This may be seen only on radiographs or not at all. The speed of spread is directly proportional to the thickness of the subcutaneous layer. Necrotizing fasciitis moves along the deep fascial plane. The overall morbidity and **mortality is 70-80%.**

Health-Care Net defines necrotizing fasciitis like this: The organisms reach the subcutaneous tissue by extension from a contiguous infection or trauma to the area, including surgery.

Dr Joseph Parazoo

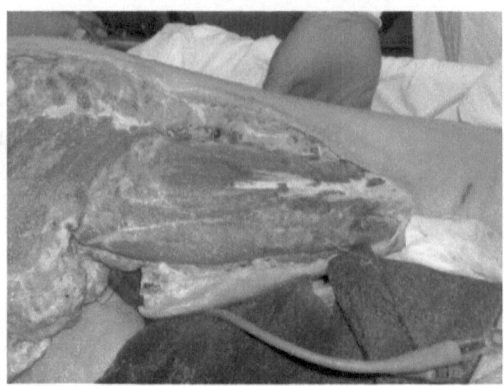

There is widespread damage to the surrounding tissue, and occlusion of small subcutaneous vessels leads to dermal gangrene. Extensive surgical incision and debridement is the mainstay of treatment, with concomitant antibiotic therapy.

There are various other necrotizing conditions that are clinically very difficult to distinguish from one another and from necrotizing fasciitis.

According to Wikipedia encyclopedia: Necrotizing fasciitis or fasciitis necroticans, commonly known as "flesh-eating bacteria," is a rare infection of the deeper layers of skin and subcutaneous tissues (fascia). Many types of bacteria can cause necrotizing fasciitis of which Group A streptococcus is the most common cause.

This disease is one of the fastest-spreading infections known as it spreads easily across the fascial plane within the subcutaneous tissue. For this reason, it is popularly called the "flesh-eating disease" and although rare, it became well-known to the public in the 1990s.

Even with topnotch care today, the prognosis can be bleak, with a mortality rate of around 25% and severe disfigurement common in survivors. Mortality is nearly 100% if

Surviving MRSA

not properly treated. In February 2004, a rarer but even more serious form of the disease has been observed in increasing frequency, with several cases found specifically in California. In these cases, the bacterium causing it was a strain of Staphylococcus aureus (i.e. Staphylococcus, not Streptococcus as stated above) which is resistant against methicillin, the antibiotic usually used for treatment.

    According to British Columbia Ministry of Health Services: Necrotizing fasciitis is a rare bacterial infection that can destroy skin and the soft tissues beneath it, including fat and the tissue covering the muscles (fascia). Because these tissues often die rapidly, a person with necrotizing fasciitis is sometimes said to be infected with "flesh-eating" bacteria, especially Streptococcus pyogenes.
    Necrotizing fasciitis is very rare but serious. There are between 90 and 200 cases per year in Canada. Many people who get necrotizing fasciitis are in good health prior to the infection.

    According to the National Necrotizing Fasciitis Foundation (NNFF): Necrotizing fasciitis is a bacterial infection. This bacteria attacks the soft tissue and the fascia, which is a sheath of tissue covering the muscle. Necrotizing fasciitis can occur in an extremity following a minor trauma, or after some other type of opportunity for the bacteria to enter the body such as surgery. In order for someone to contract Necrotizing fasciitis, the bacteria must be introduced into the body. This occurs either from direct contact with someone carrying the bacteria, or because of the bacteria is being carried by the person him or herself.
    When the infection is caused by the lightening-fast Group A Strep bacteria, the specific bacteria which causes the

Dr Joseph Parazoo

flesh-eating disease, people can go from perfectly healthy to death's door in a matter of days. Other cases of Necrotizing fasciitis, caused by a mixed bag of bacteria, can be slower moving and less deadly.

In all cases, however, prompt treatment is essential in this condition. It is one of the fastest spreading infections known, so time is the most important factor in survival.
The Group A Strep infection (flesh-eating bacteria) is most common with minor trauma. A mixed bacterial infection is often the cause after surgery.

Group A Strep is the same bacteria that causes strep throat. However, there are various strains of the bacteria, some of which are more powerful than others (with stronger m-protein serotypes). If the right set of conditions are present, this is when the necrotizing fasciitis occurs.

The name "flesh-eating bacteria" is a little sensational, but essentially, this is what the bacteria appears to do. It gets into the body, quickly reproduces, and gives off toxins and enzymes that destroy the soft tissue and fascia, which quickly becomes gangrenous (dead).

This gangrenous tissue must be surgically removed to save the life of the patient. The bacteria also stealthily hides itself from the body's innate immune system, allowing it to spread rapidly along tissue planes. Necrotizing fasciitis causes excruciating pain, dangerously low blood pressure, confusion, high fever, and severe dehydration due to the toxins poisoning the body.

Unfortunately, Necrotizing fasciitis sometimes occurs beneath the skin with few symptoms to explain the victim's symptoms. This results in a great many cases of misdiagnoses.

Surviving MRSA

Dr Joseph Parazoo

Chapter Eighteen
Fears of the Dark

Kim stirred when the nurse walked in. She walked over and picked up the IV line. She slowly inserted the needle and started to press the plunger. Kim drifted back to sleep.

A few minutes later there were four people standing around her bed as she opened her eyes. There were two nurses on each side of the bed. They were placing some kind of web belts around various areas of her body.

"Morning, Kim," one of the nurses said.

"What is going on?" Kim asked.

"We are taking you for your bath."

"What are all of these belts for?"

"Since you are not able to walk, we have to lift you out of bed," one of the nurses replied. All of the belts were snapped into place. *Vvrrrrrr...* the electric winch started to operate.

"Ahh," she gasped in fright; all the blood left her face.

"You don't have to be scared; we will make sure that you won't fall. It's okay. You are safe," one of the nurses said.

The winch continued to lift her into the air. From the corner of her eye, she could see a stainless-steel table on wheels. Then they flipped her over. Kim was in mid-air, and now looking straight down at the tile floor. "Ahh," she gasped again.

The nurses grabbed the webs and placed her on the table face-down. The nurses removed the straps and pushed her across the hall. Since she was on her stomach, she couldn't see what they were doing. The nurse turned off the

Surviving MRSA

wound-vac.

Once the suction of the machine stopped, the warmth of the blood rushed to her wound. It felt like this warm liquid covering her leg. She was startled when she felt the cool soap. This was when the blood had stabilized within her muscles. She felt the tingling run across her legs when the nurse started to pull the plastic sheeting away.

"*We need to flip her over,*" one of the nurses spoke up.

Two of the nurses rolled her onto her side. She now lay naked on this cold stainless-steel table. She started to shiver as the goose bumps ran across her skin.

This reminded her of a counter in a commercial kitchen. Looking up, she saw a water hose hanging on a hook. She was on the counter and about ready to get sprayed off. Just like you would dishes, before they go through a dishwasher. She hoped they don't put her in a dishwasher. This wasn't bad. She was getting the royal treatment, she had four nurses giving her a bath.

"*Bunt, bunt, bunt sind alle meine Kleider.*" The nurse started to sing a little song in German.

Two other nurses were washing other parts. They had adjusted the water just right. It wasn't too hot or too cold. They sprayed her down and started to carefully wash her body. They finished washing her left leg. Then one of the nurses grabbed her right leg, the one with the wound. She had a tight grip on it, when she raised it into the air.

"*Bunt, bunt, bunt ist alles, was ich hab.*" The German singing continued. As soon as the brush touched the soft raw flesh, it felt like she was stuck with a thousand needles. She just gritted her teeth.

"*Ahhhhh.*" Kim started to scream from the pain when they started to scrub.

"*Sorry. We have to do this.*" The brush started to

Dr Joseph Parazoo

loosen old scabs, dried blood, and pieces of skin.
"*Could I get some pain medication?*"
"*You have had all the pain medicine we can give you.*"
"*Bunt, bunt, bunt ist alles, was ich hab.*" The German tunes eased Kim's thoughts. One nurse tightened her grip on the leg. The nurse with the brush kept scrubbing.
"*Darum lieb ich alles, was so bunt ist.*" The German song continued.
Imagine using hard bristle brush on an open wound, pressed against the raw flesh and muscle. Now imagine that someone else is using it, where they cannot feel how much pressure they are placing on it. Sending intense pain to her brain.
She tried to shift, but I couldn't move. Not only was her muscle control impaired, there was the nurse with a tight grip. The pain was excruciating. The scrubbing continued to remove dried blood, chunks of fat, and the old useless scabs.
"*Will you quit that singing!*" one of the nurses said as she continued to scrub the brush against Kim's open leg muscle. The nurse squeezed the handle on the water hose. The rusty, muddy syrup slid down her leg.
"*Leave her alone. She is the only thing keeping me from hitting you,*" Kim commented; then she grit her teeth, and tried to bear the pain. Concentrating on the singing. The muddy sludge was washed away and ran down the drain, one more time.
"*Weil mein Schatz ein Maler, Maler ist.*" The German singer continued. The singing reminded her of the early days, when her grandma would sing to her. Her grandmother on her father's side was a full-blooded German.

Kim opened her eyes and looked around. The sun

Surviving MRSA

was shining through the window. It gave the room a nice feeling. *How did I get back in bed? The last thing I remember was resting on the table after they quit washing me.*

With the happenings of the day, Kim had a restless night. She tossed and turned, just trying to get some rest. Finally, she drifted into sleep.

The room was fairly dark, only some small night-lights in the hall. She looks around, and finds herself in a hospital. She was standing in the hallway. Straight ahead of her, at the end of the hall, there is a sign that reads "exit." She starts to walk toward it, but for some reason, she has to drag one foot. *Why doesn't my leg work?*

As she passes the room on her left, a walking brush starts to follow her. It is closing in on her as she looks over her shoulder. She passes a door on her right. She tries to speed up as another brush joins the pursuit. Before she can get halfway down the hall, something trips her. She falls flat on her stomach.

The brushes start to scrub her open wound. She tries to swat them away, but she can't get rid of them. She begins to scream. With a startle, she opens her eyes, and finds herself fighting with the sheet. After a few moments, her eyelids were too heavy to hold open. She entered the darkness one more time.

She found herself in an old apartment, and the walls were closing in. When she looked up, she saw several disfigured people, staring down at her. They started to laugh and point at her as the walls continued to close in. The room was shrinking, fast.

She ran toward the door, to run away from them.

Dr Joseph Parazoo

When she opened the door, she collided with an enormous bug. A monstrous bacteria, bigger than she was, and it obviously intended to eat her alive. Her eyes, popped open, wide. Looking around, she found nothing.

Buzz.... Buzz ...."Yes, Kim. What can I do for you?"
"I'm a little frightened."
"About what?"
"I am afraid, that I might have one of those seizures."
"Would you like me to sit in here for a while?"
"That would be nice. Thank you."

The night was calm and peaceful, at least on the outside. It was hard for her to get to sleep. The nurse could tell that Kim was having problems. She started to sing a little song in German.

"Bunt, bunt, bunt sind alle meine Kleider." This calmed Kim's nerves a little as she tried to think of her grandmother.

"Bunt, bunt, bunt ist alles, was ich hab." Kim finally drifted off to sleep with a slight smile on her face.

The sun was just starting to slip past the horizon. The sky was filled with bright blues, purples, and black. A slight breeze rustled the leaves. The family was gathered around, watching television.

Outside, she could hear the dogs, barking at the various noises and shadows. As the night continued to creep into the valley, she knew that a storm was on the way. The dogs changed their tone, and the wind began to whistle. Then suddenly, there was complete silence. The only sound to be heard was the voices from the television.

Crack. The lightning struck. *"One thousa...."* The thunder rolled across the sky.

"It's almost on top of us... Less than a half mile."

Surviving MRSA

Crackle... Rumble. The lightning and the thunder hit, almost at the same time. You could feel the house shake. Within minutes, the rain started to fall, light at first. The rain started to increase, with every minute. The rain pounded the house and ran down the roof, collecting in puddles at the edge of the house. They spent the rest of the night, in each other's arms.

    The healing process continued to undergo unseen changes. Kim hadn't thought about the bath from hell for over a week. They had been completing daily sponge baths. The nurse walked in bright and early in the morning. She walked around Kim's bed and reached for the IV. She inserted the needle into the pick line, and pushed the plunger. About a half hour later, four nurses walked into the room.
    It was time for another bath. They started to put the web belts around her.
    "Oh, goody. Do I really have to use the lift?" Kim responded rather sarcastically. The nurses looked around at each other, they all shook their heads.
    "No, I guess we don't." Since she had already had one of those baths, Kim's mind started to work. She knew what to expect. She started to feel the pain before they even reached the room. She sure hoped that gal would sing again. It did help.
    This bath time wasn't any better than the last one. There was just as much torture. She almost felt like a prisoner of war. She was sure glad that her heart was doing okay.

    "I have some bad news," the nurse commented as she walked in. It was sometime during the afternoon.
    "What is it?" Kim asked.
    "You don't get any dinner tonight. They have you

Dr Joseph Parazoo

scheduled for surgery tomorrow."
"Surgery? Why? Nobody said anything."
"The doctors looked at the pictures that we took at this morning's bath. They say that you have healed enough to get skin grafts."

Dr. Graph came in about an hour later and confirmed the progress. He took the time, to re-explain the whole process, and answer questions.

Buzz... Buzz...
"What can I do for you?" the nurse asked as she walked into Kim's room.
"I am having surgery tomorrow, and I'm a little scared."
"What kind?"
"Skin grafts."
"That's nothing to be afraid of."
"Why not?"
"That means you are getting better.... And these kind of surgeries are pretty easy."
"Maybe, they are, but I'm still a little scared."
"If you want, I can stay in here with you."
"Can you? That would be nice." The nurse walked out of the room. She shortly returned with a book. The nurse remained in the room all night, reading. Occasionally, when she heard Kim rustle restlessly, she would softly sing a German song.

"Darum lieb ich alles, was so bunt ist." Kim went back to sleep, with a slight smile.

Surviving MRSA

Dr Joseph Parazoo

Chapter Nineteen
M.R.S.A.

If you do not remember anything else from this book, please remember this phrase: **M.R.S.A.** This is a form of the Strep A... that is resistant to most antibiotics. This can and will turn into necrotizing fasciitis.

CA MRSA Hospitalizations rise 29%... A new study of U.S. data shows that in the five years that elapsed bet-ween the beginning of 2000 through the end of 2004, the number of people hospitalized for community-acquired.
MRSA infections rose by 29%. Possible explanations include greater resistance to antibiotics prescribed for outpatients, and more physician awareness of the seriousness of the infections–which leads them to recommend hospitalization, the authors said.

The Silent Spread of Hospital MRSA in the Community
Researchers from Bichat-Claude Bernard Hospital, Assistance Publique-Hopitaux de Paris determined that 191 patients (12.7%) had MRSA before they were released from the hospital. Of those carriers who were followed up on later, 75 (50.6%) had recovered from the infection within a year of being discharged from the hospital, the study found.
The 191 patients who had MRSA upon hospital discharge reported having 188 household contacts, and 36 (19.1%) of those who had contact with the MRSA carriers acquired the bug, although none developed a full-blown MRSA infection. Many people carry the bacteria that cause MRSA without actually developing the infection, researchers said.

Surviving MRSA

The fact that more patients are being released from hospitals and receiving some form of in-home care for serious illnesses that used to be treated only in hospitals appears to be increasing the risks of spreading MRSA at home.

"Patients with major health problems are increasingly discharged to home health care, which creates new opportunities for the transmission of hospital-acquired MRSA," the studies authors wrote in the journal Archives of Internal Medicine.

People who were elderly or who provided in-home medical care to infected people were more likely to acquire the MRSA bacteria from at-home contacts, the study found. Close, physical contact with infected persons, such as is necessary in administering medical treatment, appears to dramatically increase the risks of contracting MRSA from an infected person, researchers said.

Mozart 'was killed by super-bug like MRSA'

The composer's untimely death at the age of 35 has remained a mystery ever since he passed away in the early hours of 5 December 1791.

Now a group of Dutch researchers has suggested that he died from a bacterial infection spread by soldiers which was rife in Vienna at the time.

By studying the city's death register, they found that the three most common causes of death among men of his age were tuberculosis, severe weight loss and a condition called 'oedema' or 'dropsy' – an accumulation of fluids causing the body to swell up.

Mozart's symptoms match the last of the three, according to Dr Richard Zeger, from the Academic Medical Centre in Amsterdam, who said it could have been caused by a bacterial infection.

Dr Joseph Parazoo

He said: "I think you can compare this to a super-bug like MRSA or C.difficile." Eyewitnesses who saw Mozart days before he died, including his sister-in-law Sophie Haibel, said he was covered in a rash – consistent with a bacterial infection - and severely swollen - consistent with oedema or dropsy.

MRSA and Clostridium difficile kill 30,000 over five years

The number of people dying due to MRSA and Clostridium difficile fell sharply last year but the super-bug infections were still responsible for 30,000 deaths in five years, figures show.

Data from the Office for National Statistics (ONS) showed that the number of death certificates mentioning C. difficile fell by 29 per cent between 2007 and 2008, to 5,931.

This is the first year that mentions on a death certificate have fallen since records began in 1999. The number of death certificates mentioning MRSA — methicillin-resistant staphylococcus aureus — also fell by 23 per cent over the same period, to 1,230, the second year running that mentions have fallen.

The following information came from the British Broadcasting Corporation: MRSA stands for Methicillin Resistant Staphylococcus Aureus or Multiply Resistant Staphylococcus Aureus (S aureus). It is *resistant to the antibiotics* (emphasis added) usually used for S aureus.

This bacterium (bug) prefers warm, damp conditions like the nose, armpits and groin and is found all around. About one in four people carry this microbe, which does them no harm in normal circumstances, sitting there as a tenant.

Surviving MRSA

The microbe can be eradicated from these sites but in some people it will return—they seem to offer a harbor for S aureus.

They continue with: S aureus is a common cause of disease. Infections from it normally produce pus (e.g. boils), abscesses and wound infections. It can also cause pneumonia, infections of the heart valves (infective endocarditis) and particularly infections of artificial body parts (e.g. hip joints). S aureus produces an enzyme, coagulase, that walls off the infection but makes it more difficult for the white blood cells to then reach the bugs.

This is what they say about the antibiotic treatment: MRSA is a problem because it is difficult to treat. But it is no more dangerous (virulent) than common-or-garden S aureus. It requires extended treatment with antibiotics, and until recently the only effective antibiotics had to be given intravenously.

This would entail up to six weeks of hospital treatment. S aureus is usually resistant to penicillin because it produces an enzyme, betalactamase1, which destroys penicillin. Methicillin and Flucloxacillin are semi-synthetic antibiotics derived from penicillin that are resistant to the enzyme so they are effective against normal S aureus. MRSA has mutated further so the target of the penicillin has altered, so even methicillin does not work. MRSA is usually resistant to multiple antibiotics such as tetracycline, Trimethoprim and Erythromycin.

This portion of their article is what bothers me: **MRSA is created by antibiotic usage.** Contrary to news reports, many of the patients with MRSA in hospital have brought the bug in with them; this has been proven by

Dr Joseph Parazoo

swabbing patients on admission. MRSA is endemic in nursing homes.

MRSA rates are more related to overuse of antibiotics than poor hospital hygiene—the USA has a massive problem with resistant bacteria (Vancomycin-resistant enterococci as well as MRSA).

According to the same article, there is some hope: Recently, new antibiotics have been marketed to treat MRSA. Vancomycin has been the mainstay, largely superseded now by Teicoplanin. Now Synercid (Quinupristin or Dalfopristin), Daptomycin and Linezolid are all options. Linezolid works well orally, offering outpatient treatment as an option as both Vancomycin and Teicoplanin can only be given via an intravenous drip. Any artificial parts infected (e.g. hip replacements) have to be removed to eradicate the infection.

Swiss study highlights

new genetic shifts in MRSA infection

The study periods of this survey identified 292 S. aureus isolates causing BSI. Extensive molecular characterization, including genotyping as well as toxin, agr, and staphylococcal cassette chromosome content determinations, allowed us to describe epidemiological evolution in comparison to that discussed in our previous study.

Our main epidemiological observation shows that the incidence of BSI remained constant but that methicillin (meticillin)-resistant S. aureus strains with a wider variety of genetic backgrounds now harbor pyl, as has already been reported in different European countries.

Surviving MRSA

We noticed stable numbers of BSI episodes involving community-acquired methicillin-sensitive S. aureus (MSSA), whereas a drastic increase in the number of strains harboring the tst gene was recorded.

The increase in the number of tst gene-harboring strains is related to known hospital-acquired MSSA isolates and appears related to epidemic episodes in specific HCIs.

Monitoring the increase in prevalence of specific strains helps us understand where the standard precautions are not satisfactorily applied or do not efficiently prevent the spread of epidemic MSSA strains in these HCIs. The recent increases in incidence of these strains call for particular vigilance to avoid the spread of potentially virulent MSSA strains harboring the tst gene and for continuance of this strategy of BSI surveillance.

New super-bug harder to tackle than MRSA

But doctors are worried because the latest strains, known as enterobacteriaceae, produce enzymes that attack and counteract powerful antibiotics called carbapenems which the NHS relies on as its last line of defense against particularly damaging infections.

The HPA admits that tackling the threat posed by the bacteria "presents major challenges, [as most of them] are resistant to all standard intravenous antibiotics for treatment of severe infections".

John McConnell, editor of the medical journal the Lancet Infectious Diseases, said: "There's the potential for this to become a substantial problem of antibiotic resistance within UK hospitals, and there's not much we can do at the

Dr Joseph Parazoo

moment."

Compared to MRSA or C difficile or a regular pneumonia-type infection this is pretty small beer, purely in terms of the number of cases so far. But small beer is the way that things like MRSA started. These cases could be the start of what could go on to be a major cause of health care-acquired infections."

The situation is so serious that the HPA is urging pharmaceutical companies to urgently start producing drugs that are effective against these types of bacteria.

Surviving MRSA

Dr Joseph Parazoo

Chapter Twenty
Skin Grafts

Kim was finally making some progress toward recovery. She had been off all antibiotics for a while. She rarely took any pain killers. She had been eating solid food for almost two weeks. She had lost so much weight that she looked malnourished. However, she was gaining some of her weight back. The only medication that they gave her on a regular basis was insulin.

 Kim lay comfortable in her bed. She was being wheeled down the hallway. The doors of the elevator closed behind her as she entered. With a slight jerk, it started to descend. Thoughts of the last elevator ride popped into her mind. Several butterflies showed up in her stomach. She squeezed my hand as if to say,
 "Protect me." Her face started to grow pale. Within moments, there was another small jerk, the elevator stopped, and we take a hard right. Nothing happened; her worries of having a seizure passed. The butterflies flew away, and the color of her face, reappeared. The hallway was different. Damp, but comfortably cool. No longer in the well-cared-for building, we traveled inside a tunnel. We were taking an underground route from the Burn Center, to the main hospital.
 Dr. Graph was walking alongside the rest of us. He was outlining the planned surgery. He was going to use an autograft type of skin graft. He was going to use split thickness grafts, he had seen good results.

Surviving MRSA

Autografts are patches of healthy skin taken from another location on the person's body. First he would collect a graft from a donor site, most likely the same leg. In this process he would use an instrument called a dermatome, which shaves very thin slices of skin.
Split-thickness skin grafts are taken from the top layer of skin. Split-thickness skin grafts are usually 8 - 20 /1000 of an inch in thickness. The new skin will naturally grow to cover the wound made at the donor site

To ensure that the skin graft will adhere to the wound, he would debride the wound site, thoroughly cleaning it of bacteria, debris, and dead skin cells so that the skin graft will adhere to the wound. At that point he would then place the graft on the recipient site. The graft is then secured in place with sutures around the edge of the graft.
He would use ointment and mesh gauze to adhere the healthy skin surrounding the graft site. This mesh would also place pressure on the graft itself. He would then put a piece of elastic netting over the entire area. He hardly ever used casts. He liked the outcome of elastic netting. It would help keep the graft in place, and he could examine the site.
Soon we reached the operating room staging area. There was several beds. They were all waiting for their turn. The anesthesiologist was making his final preparations as Dr. Graph reassured us. The needle containing the proper dose of anesthesia was inserted into the pick line.
"I'll watch out for her," he said as he pushed the plunger. We were told that the procedure would last about three hours, and where the waiting room was located. The elevator doors closed after the bed was pushed into it.
The doors opened wide as they pushed Kim's bed into the OR. She was already having trouble keeping her eyes

Dr Joseph Parazoo

open. Her blinks were getting longer as they approached the table.

"One, two, three, and move!" was called out as they slid her onto the operating table. The bright lights straight overhead were blinding. She could barely make out the blurred outlines of people. There were two on each side, looking down on her. Gloved hands in the air, their faces covered with masks. As she went into total blackness, another figure showed up. It was Jesus, watching over the procedure.

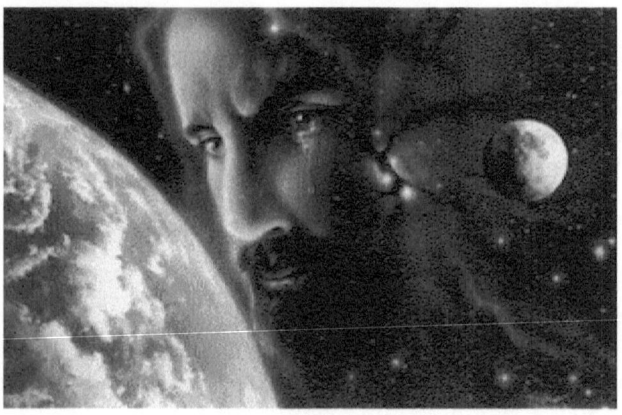

"Dermatome," he said, as he approached the operating table. An instrument resembled a large potato peeler was placed in his hand.

With precision, he removed a large section of skin from her thigh, and handed it to his assistant. Returning to remove a few more slices of her healthy skin.

His assistant took the the harvested flesh, and started the process of preparing it for transplant. First the flesh went into a machine that punched several small holes and stretched the skin.

Surviving MRSA

Once the skin was reshaped and perforated, it was placed in a vat filled with life giving plasma. One slice after another, the skin was being conditioned

The graft is initially nourished by a process called plasmatic imbibition in which the graft literally "drinks plasma." New blood vessels begin growing from the recipient area into the transplanted skin within thirty-six hours in a process called capillary inosculation.

"*Re-drape,*" he commanded, handing the dermatome back to the scrub nurse and stepped away from the table. He doffed his gloves, and put on a fresh pair. The harvesting was complete, now to start the repairs.

"*Scalpel,*" he said as he placed his palm upward. The scalpel was immediately placed in his hand. With the scalpel in hand, he carefully cleaned off the jagged edges of the wound.

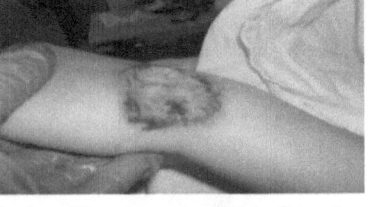

"*Suction,*" he commanded as he removed his hands from the wound area. The scrub nurse was ready, and guided the suction tube over the open wound. The machine gurgled as the rusty blood and pieces of dead flesh traveled through the plastic hose.

"Suture," He poked the curved suture needle through the edges of the skin, and drew the thread tight. He continued to secure the graph in place.

Dr Joseph Parazoo

"Scalpel," With the scalpel in hand, he carefully cleaned off the jagged edges of the wound.

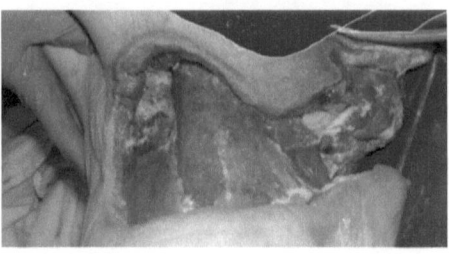

"Graph," he called stepping away from the operating table. He removed his gloves and put on a clean pair. The assistant positioned a piece of the harvested skin over the wound area.

"Suture," He poked the curved suture needle through the edges of the skin, and drew the thread tight. He continued to secure the graph in place.

"Reposition," he barked, and stepped away from the table. The scrub nurse glanced up and noticed the sweet drops forming on his forehead. Using a sterile cloth, she wiped it dry.

He had completed the procedure on the front side. He was waiting for the team to reposition her, so he could start on the biggest area.

Surviving MRSA

"Scalpel," With the scalpel in hand, he carefully cleaned off the jagged edges of the wound.

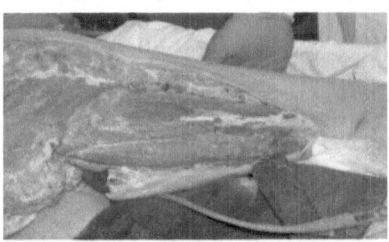

"Suction," he commanded as he removed his hands from the wound area. The scrub nurse guided the suction tube over the open wound. The machine gurgled as the rusty blood and pieces of dead flesh traveled through the plastic hose.
"Graph," he called once more, stepping away from the operating table. He removed his gloves and put on a clean pair. While the assistant positioned a piece of the harvested skin over the wound area.
"Suture," He poked the curved suture needle through the edges of the skin, and drew the thread tight. He continued to secure the graph in place.

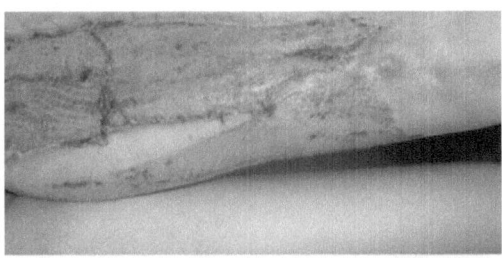

"Graph," he called once more, stepping away from

the operating table. The assistant positioned a piece of the harvested skin over the wound area.

"Suture," He poked the curved suture needle through the edges of the skin, and drew the thread tight. He continued to secure the graph in place.

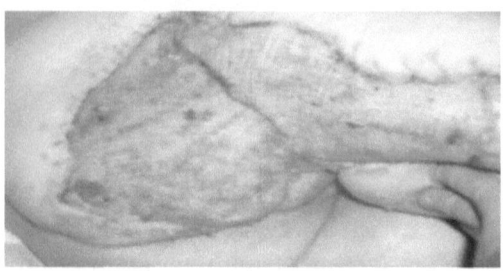

"Graph," he called once more, stepping away from the operating table. The assistant placed another piece of the harvested skin over the wound area.

"Suture," He poked the curved suture needle through the edges of the skin, and drew the thread tight. He continued to secure the graph in place.

The final stitch was made. Dr. Graph left the operating room, stripping off his gloves and gown as he went. He proceeded to the locker room for a cup of coffee.

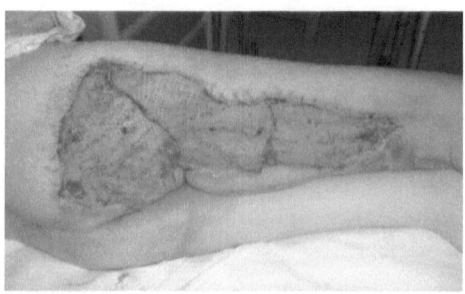

Surviving MRSA

The assistant placed ointment and mesh gauze to adhere the healthy skin surrounding the graft site. The nurses would finish cleaning the area. Then the bandage her up.

We just sat silently as she lay in bed. Me in the chair, holding her hand. As the time went by, we closed our eyes, our heads tilted back.
Listening to the silence. The sunlight turned amber, and then a muddy orange, beyond the large window. Slowly, the room filled up with shadows. She slept and dreamed.

The sky was bright blue, it was golden and fuzzy around the edges. She was naked with Joe, lying in a meadow where the grass felt like feathers. High above the world, a meadow atop a towering pillar of rock. There was a warm wind that was cleaner than sunshine. An eagle drifted by and started to circle. It was just drifting and gliding on the warm currents, as if protecting them.

We were able to start the "walking" process, two days after the surgery. They brought in a recliner, for her to use. We were told not to overdo it. That she would get tired very fast. That she would have to build the muscles up.
Every day, we would help Kim perform various exercises. She didn't have too much of a problem sitting up. Once it came to using her leg muscles, then she needed a little support.
When she first stood on her feet, she felt unstable. She said it was as if she was a tree in a wind storm. There wasn't much strength, and she was a little wobbly. As she tried to take her first step, nothing was working right.
"It seems like the connection from my brain to my feet

Dr Joseph Parazoo

is missing. My brain tells my foot to move, but it won't listen," she commented.

"*Don't worry about lifting the foot. Just try and slide it a little ways."* She concentrated and was able to slide her left foot about the length of her foot. I continued to face her, holding on to both arms.

"*Now, try to stand up straight."* She put her mind to it, and stood taller. She seemed to be in a hurry to move the other foot as she slid it forward.

"*You're doing good.... Let's try another step."* We went through the whole process again. Slide the left foot, stand tall, then slide the right foot.

"*You just let me know when you want to stop,"* I said. Before long, we were standing next to the window, which was about twelve feet away from the bed. I was proud of Kim for walking so far on her first try.

"*I would like to rest for a few minutes,"* she said as she tried to catch her breath. She just stood by the window, enjoying the green grass and bushes.

"*It won't be long, and I will be...out there,"* she commented. After about five minutes, once she was comfortably rested, we repeated the entire process, back to the bed.

"*Not only are my legs tired, so is my mind, from all the concentration,"* she commented. Shortly after that, she was peacefully sleeping.

The tendons and muscles were hard to command. We made several trips from one end of the room to the other. She wanted out of that room.

The next day, we took most of the walks up and down the hallways. Whenever anyone was in the room, she wanted to go for a walk. A continuous thought ran through her mind;

Surviving MRSA

The sooner I can build up my strength, the sooner I can go home. We would grab the walker and keep her steady.

Once she got moving, it was hard to stop her. She kept pushing herself. She tried all kind of things to coax her legs and feet to work right. It wasn't long before she started to pick her feet up off of the floor. Within two days, she could walk outside.

Kim's abilities were increasing at great speed. She was moving around pretty good. She didn't really require a lot of attention. They decided that the room we were in could be better used by a more critical patient.

This room was closer to the outside garden area, which she liked. They also transferred the recliner. She was more than happy to spend more time in the chair. Since she was more or less mobile, she felt more independent about everything.

Buzz... Buzz... Kim pushed the button for a little help.
"What can I do for you, Kim?" the nurse asked as he walked into the room.
"I feel funny."
"What do you mean, you feel funny?"

Feeling dizzy, poor concentration, tremors of hands, and sweating are common symptoms of hypoglycemia. Hypoglycemia is the term doctors use for low blood sugar. You can faint or have a seizure if blood sugar level gets too low. The normal range of the blood sugar levels is between 85 and 105.

"Something is wrong. I think my blood sugar is low."
"I don't think so... It's not time to check, but we can check it, anyway," he said as he reached for the glucose tester.

Dr Joseph Parazoo

"Thirty-six. That is quite low. Let me get you something to eat." He walked out of the room, thinking, *Wow, a blood sugar level of twenty-seven would have put her into a coma.*

Once he was out of the room, sort of in a panic, he scrambled to find some food. It wasn't very long before he returned. He gave her a tall glass of orange juice, chocolate pudding, and some graham crackers.

He grabbed a chair and sat alongside of her. While she ate, he began to think. *It's only 2:30 in the morning.* About a half hour later, he re-checked her blood sugar. *"You are safe now. You're at ninety-two. Next time, I'll believe you."*

"Congratulations.... You have graduated," he said as he handed her a black metal, adjustable cane. *"Try using this."* Kim smiled as she reached for the cane. She was glad to get rid of that walker.

It was a nice sunny day, with a slight wind. Today was the day. Dr. Graph had told us that almost one hundred percent of the skin graft took. The date was February twenty-eighth. The last day of the month.

Seventy to eighty percent of those people that are diagnosed with necrotizing fasciitis die. Of the remaining twenty percent, seventy percent of them lose at least one limb. The best part of it, Kim was able to walk out of the hospital. Sure, she used the cane, but it was all under her own power.

Do we feel lucky? You're damn right we do.

"Since this is your day, what would you like to do first?"

"I want the top down, and a mocha," she responded. I pushed the button, and the black canvas top of the convertible folded down. There was an espresso shop just down the road.

Surviving MRSA

Dr Joseph Parazoo

Chapter Twenty One
Treatment

What's the likely outcome? Anywhere from minimal scars to death and everywhere in between. For those lucky enough to survive most often at least some removal of skin is required. Often this requires skin grafting. Amputation is sometimes needed to remove the affected limb. Legs, hands, fingers, toes, arms, have all been sacrificed to save the life of NF patients.

The British Broadcasting Corporation explains it this way: Aggressive combination regime antibiotics therapy—A broad spectrum of drugs will be used, including Cefazolin, clindamycin, gentamycin, penicillin and metronidazole. However, because antibiotics therapy sometimes does not work, doctors are pressured to either prevent shock from happening at all, or to catch it in the early— and more easily treatable—stages. If the bacteria in the bloodstream have reached dangerously high levels, antibiotics therapy can actually do the patient harm rather than good. Therefore, scientists have been working to develop drugs to stop the cascade of events that cause damage to the blood vessels and organs.

Theoretically, antibiotics therapy combined with anti-inflammatory drugs should be effective in treating all but the worst of septic shock cases; however, these anti-inflammatory drugs may actually worsen the patient's condition because they further suppress the patient's immune system and

Surviving MRSA

increase the risk of secondary infections. Monoclonal antibodies against LPS (Lipopolysaccharide - which causes septic shock) have been raised and tested, but therapy using these antibodies must be carried out very early in the shock process to have any positive effect.

Other therapies that have been developed—those directed against TNF and other shock-related cytokines—are too expensive (at least $2500 per treatment course) to be of any practical value.

Surgical debridement—i.e. cutting away dead or infected tissue, or removal of foreign matter from the flesh. This involves surgical excision and drainage to remove all infected, necrotic tissue and fascia until clean, healthy, pearly gray fascia is identified in all margins of the wound.

This will be carried out as soon as the patient is diagnosed with necrotizing fasciitis to prevent further spreading of the disease. If diagnosed early, tissue loss can be relatively small—only flesh, subcutaneous tissue and fat will be removed. If the disease is allowed to progress, however, amputation of affected limbs may be necessary if the victim is to survive.

Treatment may also include usage of a hyperbaric oxygen chamber—This is to increase the partial pressure of oxygen in the blood, thus enabling wounds to heal better by reducing oedema due to vasoconstriction of the arterioles and hypoxia. The white blood cells are also strengthened in their ability to fight the invading bacteria. However, this treatment is more commonly used in the case of gas gangrene, which is typically caused by Clostridium perfringens.

Dr Joseph Parazoo

These are only essential treatment measures; however, because of the complication of necrotizing fasciitis, subsidiary patient management is needed to deal with the excruciating pain experienced by patients during dressing changes, and to encourage the body to heal.

The caloric intake of patients recovering from massive trauma is usually increased twofold or threefold, often with dietetic recommendations by a dietitian. The emotional trauma suffered by the patients due to pain, severe disfigurement following surgery, and intense emotions must also be handled to ensure complete recovery.

Health-Care Net has these words: Treatment of necrotizing fasciitis is most effective if the infection is recognized in time. Antibiotics and surgical removal of dead tissue are required. If the tissue destruction is widespread, extensive surgery or amputation might be the only way to prevent death.

While early diagnosis and treatment are the key to preventing devastating tissue destruction, physicians and patients often fail to recognize necrotizing fasciitis and its severity. Being rare, and with an onset that resembles flu-like symptoms, it is often missed until the infection has advanced.

One alerting sign is unusually severe pain—far greater than normal for a cut or wound—and painful lymph nodes. For example, a cut on the toe or a surgical leg wound, followed some hours later by severe pain either in the toe, leg, or in the groin (as the infection travels to the lymph nodes), can warn of this potentially deadly, fast-spreading infection.

How manuka honey helps fight infection

Manuka honey may kill bacteria by destroying key

Surviving MRSA

bacterial proteins. Dr Rowena Jenkins and colleagues from the University of Wales Institute – Cardiff investigated the mechanisms of manuka honey action and found that its anti-bacterial properties were not due solely to the sugars present in the honey.

The work was presented this week 7-10 September, at the Society for General Microbiology's meeting at Heriot-Watt University, Edinburgh.Meticillin resistant Staphylococcus aureus MRSA was grown in the laboratory and treated with and without manuka honey for four hours. The experiment was repeated with sugar syrup to determine if the effects seen were due to sugar content in honey alone. The bacterial cells were then broken and the proteins isolated and separated on a system that displayed each protein as an individual spot.

Many fewer proteins were seen from the manuka honey-treated MRSA cells and one particular protein, FabI, seemed to be completely missing. FabI is a protein that is needed for fatty acid biosynthesis. This essential process supplies the bacteria with precursors for important cellular components such as lipopolysaccarides and its cell wall. The absence of these proteins in honey-treated cells could help explain the mode of action of manuka honey in killing MRSA.

Crises Occur Due To Lack Of Use Of Sun Energy

"The biggest setback we have encountered is lack of immunity. Most of us suffer from poor immunity. We have no energy to tackle day-to-day living. We can overcome all this by taking sun energy. It is an established fact that total health includes — mental, physical, **and spiritual wellness.**"

If you spend your days indoors, you miss the ultraviolet (UV) component of sunlight. Glass removed the UV component. The glass bulbs of light bulbs absorb UV. If you try to grow

Dr Joseph Parazoo

plants under incandescent bulbs, they will die.

If you work in an office or factory setting, be aware that fluorescent lighting increases fatigue and drains you of vitamin A and energy. Studies have proven that UV light lowers the blood sugar of diabetics.

When the blood sugar drops, people run out of energy, become irritable, drowsy, and emotional. Exposure to sunlight raises insulin level and lowers blood sugar. Sunlight entering the eyes provides a counterbalance to blood sugar lowering effect of sunlight hitting the skin.

Surviving MRSA

Dr Joseph Parazoo

Chapter Twenty Two
Preventing

For the most part, there is no way to prevent the bacteria from being around. What a person has to do is make sure that they take care of any wound. The strep A bacteria lives in and on people. There are a few things that I would suggest;

1) Eat right, so that your immune system is good.

2) If you work around a lot of people, take a shower when you get off work.

3) Don't get all "freaked out" about this stuff, and use common sense.

4) If you happen to receive any wounds, take care of them; they will not just go away.

5) People with strep throat should stay home and away from others.

According to the CDC: The spread of all types of Group A Strep infection can be reduced by good hand washing, especially after coughing and sneezing and before preparing foods or eating. Persons with sore throats should be seen by a doctor who can perform tests to find out whether the illness is strep throat. If the test result shows strep throat, the person should stay home from work, school, or day care until

Surviving MRSA

24 hours after taking an antibiotic.
All wounds should be kept clean and watched for possible signs of infection such as redness, swelling, drainage, and pain at the wound site. A person with signs of an infected wound, especially if fever occurs, should seek medical care. It is not necessary for all persons exposed to someone with an invasive group A strep infection (i.e. necrotizing fasciitis or strep toxic shock syndrome) to receive antibiotic therapy to prevent infection. However, in certain circumstances, antibiotic therapy may be appropriate. That decision should be made after consulting with your doctor.

   The British Broadcast Corporation reports this information: Recently, however, it has been established that the usage of pain-relieving non-steroidal anti-inflammatory drugs (such as ibuprofen) greatly increases the risk of developing necrotizing fasciitis, especially among children with varicella-zoster virus infection (aka chickenpox). Because these drugs prevent inflammation, which is important for fighting microbes, it also messes up the body's defense mechanism, thus causing multiple organ system failure.

   Health-Care Net gives the following advice: The spread of all types of GAS infection can be reduced by thorough hand washing, especially after coughing, sneezing, after caring for persons with wounds or "strep throat," before preparing foods and before eating. Both the organism and the patient susceptibility likely play a role in the development of the infection. While most group A streptococci cause only mild infections (e.g., "strep throat") some types may cause more severe disease. One factor that may be linked to the development of necrotizing fasciitis is the production of proteases (enzymes that break down proteins) by some group

Dr Joseph Parazoo

A streptococci.
Susceptibility of the individual is also important. Investigation of family clusters has shown that the same type of bacteria can cause severe illness in one family member and only mild or no illness in others.

Fresh Air to Prevent MRSA....

For those looking for a more practical way to avoid viruses such as the H1N1 strain of flu, MRSA or C difficile, Macdonald claims to have the answer. "It was always a mystery why in field hospitals there were relatively low rates of infection among patients," says Macdonald.

"Remember that in the past we used to wheel out hospital patients to aid recuperation, but we don't anymore. Based on research developed at the Government's Porton Down facility in the 1960s, we realized that the answer was rather simple."

Dubbed the "open-air factor" by the original researchers, the science centers on the hydroxyl radical compound, naturally created in the open air when ozone merges with olefins, a type of carbon molecule. This mixture acts as a natural disinfectant against pathogens or germs that lurk in the atmosphere.

Putting this science to work, Mid-States has launched AD – Atmospheric Disinfection – a machine that helps to mimic the infection-busting characteristics of the outside, indoors. "You could argue you could do exactly the same thing with a 14-pound sledge hammer and take the windows out," says Macdonald. "And it would work because as a species we haven't adapted to working in enclosed spaces. We've only been inside for 20 or so generations and we haven't fully adapted that quickly."

Standing about 2ft tall, the AD looks like an innocuous heater plugged into a wall. It spews hydroxyl radicals into the air which collide with harmful pathogens, without any noise, smell or color.

Surviving MRSA

Crises Occur Due To Lack Of Use Of Sun Energy

"The biggest setback we have encountered is lack of immunity. Most of us suffer from poor immunity. We have no energy to tackle day-to-day living. We can overcome all this by taking sun energy. It is an established fact that total health includes — mental, physical, **and spiritual wellness.**"

If you spend your days indoors, you miss the ultraviolet (UV) component of sunlight. Glass removed the UV component. The glass bulbs of light bulbs absorb UV. If you try to grow plants under incandescent bulbs, they will die. If you grow your plants under full spectrum light, they will flourish. Some plants, such as trees, need the light of the sun. You can keep trees inside for short periods of time, but you will notice a significant increase in vigor and growth if you put the trees out in the sunlight.

If you work in an office or factory setting, be aware that fluorescent lighting increases fatigue and drains you of vitamin A and energy. Studies have proven that UV light lowers the blood sugar of diabetics (Pincussen cited in **(Sunlight.as.ro,2005)**. When the blood sugar drops, people run out of energy, become irritable, drowsy, and emotional.

Exposure to sunlight raises insulin level and lowers blood sugar. Sunlight entering the eyes provides a counterbalance to blood sugar lowering effect of sunlight hitting the skin (Relkin cited in **(Sunlight.as.ro, 2005)**. The sun gazing guru, HRM, sleeps for a couple of hours per day and feels little or no fatigue.

The ancient civilizations worshiped the sun and used the sun's energy to heal their bodies. As we get closer to the modern civilization, we see individuals who do not get enough sunlight.

Some of the people work in environments where sunlight is absent. Others stay out of sunlight for fear of developing

Dr Joseph Parazoo

cancer. As the research into vitamin D is accumulating, it's hard to know where the accolades should start. "Activated vitamin D is one of the most potent inhibitors of cancer cell growth," says Michael F. Holick, PhD, MD, who heads the Vitamin D, Skin, and Bone Research Laboratory at Boston University School of Medicine. "It also stimulates your pancreas to make insulin. It regulates your immune system."

What is better than free? If it is also highly effective, then that is surely better!

Vitamin D is a fat-soluble vitamin that is used by the body in the absorption of calcium. Sunshine is a significant source of vitamin D. The body can produce vitamin D after exposure to ultraviolet (UV) rays from the sun. UV rays from sunlight trigger vitamin D synthesis in your skin.

A deficiency of vitamin D can occur when individuals have limited exposure to sunlight. Vitamin D deficiency can lead to rickets and osteomalacia. Rickets results in soft bones and skeletal deformities. Osteomalacia results in muscular weakness and weak bones.

"What's really remarkable is that vitamin D deficiency is epidemic throughout the entire United States, through all age groups. And I'll give you some examples. It's well known that elders throughout the United States are at high risk. And upwards of 40-60% are at risk for vitamin D deficiency.

"But we also now realize that even younger adults that are otherwise active and who may be always wearing screen before they go outdoors, or they never see the light of day because they're **working all the time.**

Surviving MRSA

Dr Joseph Parazoo

Chapter Twenty Three
Rehabilitation

Now the road to recovery began. We were no longer in the hospital, but we were not through with the doctors. We had to see a diabetic specialist. We had to have several follow-ups, just to make sure that I was taking care of her right. We had to go back in about a month to remove the colostomy bag. If everything went right...then just maybe.

The strength of Kim's muscles continued to improve. We would go for walks every day. Each day we would walk a little further. Every time that I would change her bandages, I would examine the area for signs "that didn't look right." If I ever had any questions or concerns, I would call the Burn Center for instructions.

Kim was started out with thirty-five units of Humulin N every morning, and fifteen units at night. We worked out a sliding scale, of the amount of insulin to take, at what sugar level. This is when she would have to use Humulin R insulin.

> Humulin N, also known as NPH, is called an intermediate acting insulin. Upon injection, it starts to release the active ingredients on a upward trend. It reaches its peak about five hours later. The remaining ingredients are released in a tapered-off trend, until they are gone. It can last from twelve to twenty-four hours.

There were several reasons that we wanted to stay on the injectable insulin. One reason is the insurance company. We knew that they would pay for the testing supplies. On the

Surviving MRSA

injectable type of insulin, you are allowed testing five or six times a day. If you were on the oral type of medication, they stopped at two or three times a week.

> Humulin R, also known as regular insulin, starts to work immediately upon injection. All of the active ingredients are usually dispensed into the bloodstream within four hours. It can last up to twelve hours.

If you only test your blood sugar level a couple of times a week how can you really regulate it? Another main reason was that we figured that a person would have a lot more control of how much medication they took. Sure, it is a hassle to test your blood several times a day.
However, if you start to feel a little weird, you can test. In order for you to properly "control" this disease, you have to change your diet. How would a person know which foods did what, if you did not test? We had also heard many stories about people that had been on the oral type medications. We didn't want to deal with anything else unexpected.

One thing we didn't want to do was go back to the hospital. If we wanted to get rid of this colostomy bag, we had to. We walked into the Emanuel Hospital with apprehension. It wasn't too long before she was in the all-too-familiar gown. She lay on the bed, just waiting. This surgery and little stay was more or less our choice. She wasn't really sick this time. We knew what to expect. One of the assisting doctor came out and introduced himself. He was looking over the records.
"So, we are doing a colostomy reversal. And, putting a skin graft on the right wrist," he commented.
"Hey, wait a minute. You have the wrong hand. Who

Dr Joseph Parazoo

did you say you were?"
"I am assisting Dr. Graph."
"You better get this right. I've heard of those kind of horror stories. She doesn't need any wrong surgeries today! Why don't you get a marker to remind yourself!" Just about that time, the anesthesiologist walked over.
"Are you allergic to any medication?" he asked.
"Yeah, she had seizures with one, but we don't know the name of it."
"I'll be back in a few minutes," he said as he walked away. Within a few minutes, he was reading through her records. He started to prepare the anesthesia.
The bed was wheeled down the hallway. Within minutes, Kim's eyes started to blink rapidly as she fought the urge. The doors swung wide as the bed crashed into them. She could barely make out the figures. Her blinks were getting longer, harder to hold her eyes open.

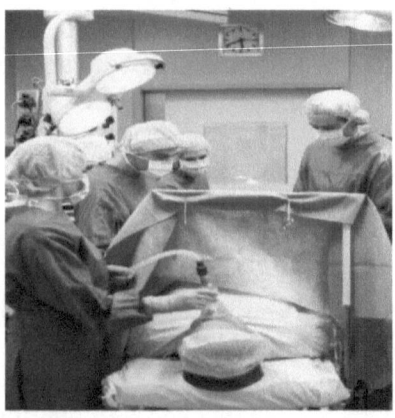

"How are you doing, Kim?" Dr. Graph said. She started to drift, with the thought, *That voice. It sounds familiar.... It's Dr. Graph.* A slight smile appeared on her face

Surviving MRSA

as she went completely under.

Over the past month and a half, she had been seen by many doctors. She didn't remember and never met most of them. But she did like Dr. Graph. He was about our age. He wasn't tall, but he was dark and handsome. He projected a certain air, and his crew respected him.

Many didn't care for his stern attitude of perfection; he was hard on them. But, when it came to the patients, he was gentle and kind. He took the time to explain things, and didn't look down on them.

This isn't near as demanding as his normal surgeries. He specialized in the invasive and radical debridement, skin grafts, and dealing with burn victims. He spent many hours under that bright light, looking over the surgical mask. The surgeries were grueling, and not always positive. But, he enjoyed the contribution that he could make. This was a simple colostomy reversal. He could do it with his eyes closed.

The overhead lights had already been focused on the patient's lower abdomen. Blue surgical drapes were clamped in place, framing a rectangle of exposed skin. A colostomy is a surgical procedure that involves connecting a part of the colon onto the anterior abdominal wall, leaving the patient with an opening on the abdomen called a stoma. This opening is formed from the end of the large intestine drawn out through the incision and sutured to the skin.

"Scalpel," he said as he extended his hand palm upward. He made a delicate incision where the sutures used to be, as he slowly removed the colostomy bag from her warm intestines.

"Suture," He poked the curved suture needle through the edge of the colon, and drew the thread tight.

Dr Joseph Parazoo

After a colostomy, feces leave the patient's body through the stoma, and collect in a pouch attached to the patient's abdomen which is changed when necessary. People with colostomies must wear an external pouch to collect intestinal waste.

Ostomy pouches fit close to the body and are usually not visible under regular clothing unless the wearer allows the pouch to become too full. Modern pouches are made of lightweight plastic and are attached to the skin with an adhesive wafer made of pectin or similar organic material.

The wafer is cut with a hole to fit snugly around the base of the stoma to prevent leakage of stool onto the skin (and consequent skin irritation).

Ordinarily the pouch must be emptied several times a day. Many people find it convenient to do this whenever they make a trip to the bathroom to urinate. This bag would be changed every two to five days, when the wafer starts to deteriorate. Or, when you have an explosion and the bag flies across the room.

"Retract," Dr. Graph said as he snipped the needle and tied the last stitch. The scrub nurse took hold of the stainless-steel retractors and gently tugged the wound open.

He gently pushed the exposed intestines back in place. He reached in to make sure there weren't any kinks. He forgot how warm and slippery the intestines could be. What a wondrous sensation, to be cradled in the heat of the human body. It was like being welcomed back into the womb.

"Suture," He poked the curved suture needle through the edge of the skin, and drew the thread tight. One more stitch, and this operation will be over.

Surviving MRSA

"You're not Brad Pitt," Kim said when she opened her eyes.

"No, I'm not," the anesthesiologist said as he chuckled. We began the underground trek towards the burn ward. We were assigned one of the small rooms, waiting for the time to leave. We were expecting the stay to be only a couple of days.

Placing the cold stethoscope on Kim's belly, Dr. Graph listened... *"That's what I wanted to hear,"* he said, with a smile on his face. *"I'll make sure that you get something to eat tomorrow. You have a good night."*

It was evening when Dr. Graph walked into the room. He checked the bandage and the wound on her stomach. *"It looks like it's coming along fine."*

"When do you think we could go home?"

"You have been taking care of her steady for the last month. Plus my crew have other people to look at. Your grafts are looking good. Your stomach wound is looking fine. Do you think that you can handle this wound?" he pointed to her stomach.

A couple of weeks went by. The wound on her stomach was almost closed up. I started to notice that she was picking her left foot really high in the air. Upon closer observation, I noticed that she was not bending her ankle. During one of the follow-ups, we discussed it with Dr. Graph. He watched Kim walk around the room for a few moments.

"It looks like you have drop foot," he said.

"What is that?"

Dr. Graph started to explain. Drop foot is a term that describes an abnormal neuromuscular (nerve and muscle)

Dr Joseph Parazoo

disorder that affects the patient's ability to raise their foot at the ankle.

Patients with drop foot usually exhibit an exaggerated or high-stepping walk. Often drop foot is caused by injury to the peroneal nerve deep within the lumbar and sacral spine. The peroneal nerve is a division of the sciatic nerve. The peroneal nerve runs along the outside of the lower leg (below the knee) and branches off into each ankle, foot, and first two toes. It innervates or transmits signals to muscle groups responsible for ankle, foot, and toe movement and sensation.

"How could that have happened, to cause this?"
"It could have happened during any of the surgeries, due to the positions that you had to be in. The peroneal nerve is susceptible to different types of injury. Some of these include nerve compression from lumbar disc herniation. Depending on the cause, drop foot may be temporary or permanent. You should have it checked out."
We decided to start with the chiropractor that we had seen before. Dr. Bones had a small office located in Newberg. Her practice could have grown over the years, if it weren't for her dislike of big business. She didn't like how they shuffled the patients through like cattle. She preferred to stay small and provide quality.
After her examination, Dr. Bones confirmed that Kim did have drop foot. *"Your hip is out of place. I found L4, L5, S1, out. We can work on that. In the meantime, you need a Orthosis brace."*
We continued to visit the chiropractor every two weeks. The brace came in, and Kim had to learn how to walk in a different way.

Surviving MRSA

Dr. General Physician said as she handed us a prescription sheet with the name of a sports injury clinic.

The sports clinic was located in McMinnville. A small waiting room, four exam-type rooms, and an exercise room.

"We assign one, maybe two therapists to each customer. We find that the sessions work out better that way. The patient feels more comfortable too. They don't have to re-explain all the problems or areas."

That sounded pretty good. The consult consisted of a small exam of the problem area. We covered the basic concerns and desired outcome. A basic outline of treatment was agreed on.

The first four sessions included heat pads to loosen up the muscles. They also performed a localized massage of the lower back and hip. They used a ultrasonic massaging tool to increase the depth. After about a half hour, we would move out to the exercise room. They showed us some specialized exercises to perform. There were various machines to help with the problem areas. However, so far, we had seen four different therapists.

The next three sessions, we saw another three different therapists. They skipped all of the prep. There was no more heat pads, no more massages, no more concern for that part of the body. We were taken straight to the exercise room.

"If this is all they are going to do, why should we pay them? We can do this at home." After we completed the workout, we walked out, never to return. We wondered, why did we have a different person for each session? They did say that there were better results, when only one or two therapists were used.

There were two things that entered our minds. One was that they couldn't stand the sight of her scars. The second was they were afraid that they might catch whatever she had.

Dr Joseph Parazoo

During one the follow-ups, Kim voiced her concerns about going back to work. She wasn't sure where or how she contracted this bacteria. She explained to Dr. Graph how she had been working on a clogged drain the week before all this happened.
"*You could have caught this anywhere. There are all types of bacteria everywhere. You can find bacteria in your home. You can find bacteria in the grocery store...actually, anywhere people are, you will find bacteria.*"
"*I'm still worried, about catching it again.*"
"*You can't live in a bubble, Kim.*" Dr. Graph gave Kim the consent to go back to work.

The first couple of weeks back to work were difficult. She would come home and complain. She was getting tired of the questions. The people didn't understand. She hated all the little comments. If she did tell them that she had necrotizing fasciitis, they would back away as if they were afraid of catching it.

Her legs were completely fatigued. She had been running off pure determination and adrenalin. Her left foot hurt because of the brace. This brace was made of plastic and only under half of her foot. She wanted to get rid of it. She barely got through eating dinner and she was ready to go to bed. I couldn't blame her; she had gone through a lot.

The brace from the chiropractor was awkward and it hurt Kim's foot. Besides that, it wasn't exercising the foot. It kept the foot flat, and wouldn't allow for any movement. This Orthosis brace could be picked up almost anywhere, for $29.95.

Kim was searching the internet, learning about the drop foot syndrome, when she found a company. We had to provide the shoes, they would create the brace, according to

Surviving MRSA

the measurements that they sent them. This one had elastic straps attached to the shoe. She would then have to operate her foot as normal. However, the straps would pull the foot upwards, so that she would not trip. This custom-made brace was only $400.

Over the months, Kim had tried to go without her brace as much as possible. By November 2005, she no longer wore the brace except at work, she was afraid that she would trip. She kept wearing the brace there, until September 2006. received were worthless.

Occasionally, I get kicked in the middle of the night. Kim experiences electrical surges through her right leg. We believe that they are just a symptoms of the body trying to rebuild the nervous system. We keep up on vitamins and minerals, plenty of exercise, and massages. She has learned and practices meditation; she says that this works.

With Kim being in the hospital for such a long time, our financial status started to suffer. Without going into great detail, and make this section shorter, we ended up at a hard spot. Our house was about to be foreclosed on. We arranged for an auction company to sell all of our stuff. We took a few essentials and keepsakes, and moved.

What a change, going from a three-bedroom house, to a one bedroom apartment. From a forty-two-inch television, to a nineteen-inch. From a three-piece leather sectional, to a couple of overstuffed chairs. Going from four vehicles, to one. Etc. Once in a while, we think about our losses, and remind ourselves it was only stuff... We were able to keep the most important thing....

Kim's life and our marriage intact.

Dr Joseph Parazoo

Surviving MRSA

Dr Joseph Parazoo

Chapter Twenty Four
Transformation

The long road to recovery for Kim begins. It was my duty to take care of her and I placed her needs above mine. The more that I provided Kim with loving care, the more relaxed I felt. I tried not to let all of my worldly problems stand in the way. It is hard to explain, but I felt softer inside.

It's about four in the morning. I'm dosing. It's pitch black. There is a shimmer of light from the stars. I find myself looking for something. It's terribly important to find it, but I don't know what it is. I'm looking in empty rooms and through doors that lead nowhere. Occasionally, I glimpse something in the shadows. A frantic -- yet hopeless -- search for that which I have lost. It is now six in the morning. I'm awake, grunting and tussling with the tangled sheets.

Realizing that doctors were only human, I wonder if it was the prayer that I made, that actually made all of the difference. It would only be fair of me at least to thank this God, for saving Kim's life.

Ah Ha! *"If I am willing to give credit to an Entity, that people call God; then I must have some belief, that this God exists. And, if this God exists, then I want to know more about this concept, called God. What is the purpose of God? What is the truth? If God exists, He should fulfill*

Surviving MRSA

the promises that are mentioned in the Bible." I remembered the following quote.

Jesus said: "Ask, and it shall be given; seek, and ye shall find; knock, and it shall be opened unto you:" (Matthew 7:7)

"*I have a lot of questions. Where do I start? If I am ever to know the 'Truth,' why not go to the Source?*" I made a very "heart felt" prayer. The first part of the prayer was to thank Him for saving Kim. The second part was accepting that God existed. The third part was for guidance, to know the truth. ......

Within seconds, a very strange feeling went through my entire body. This feeling is very hard to explain. Unless you have gone through something similar, it's hard to comprehend.

This feeling started at the top of my head, went "through" my body, all the way to my toes. It was like a wave of warm water, only in the form of energy. It was an electric surge, yet it moved very slowly. Almost as if some one -- or some thing -- was "entering" my body. It didn't hurt. It didn't startle me. Actually it felt very comforting.

There was a "calming" -- yet "uplifting" effect. The feeling was "soothing." Like a mothers touch, filled with love. My mind was very relaxed, as if there was no reason to hurry. However, there was so much "charge," I felt "all hyped up."

I hope that you have the idea. I would sum it up like this: **AWESOME!!!!**

Dr Joseph Parazoo

One of my dreams....... I was on a guided tour of a natural preserve. You know the type. You are among a group of people. The tour guide explains the sites, or teachings, as directed by the manager. They basically use a script hardly ever deviating from it. No real question and answer period.

About half way through the tour I hear; *"You would learn and understand more if you left the group, to follow your own path."*

Metaphysical Psychology

So, what is metaphysical psychology? If you ask the average person, he would probably say it was something mystic, or it has to do with "getting into someone's head."
There are many definitions of metaphysics, all valid; but for my purpose, it deals with cosmic laws and principles, and unseen forces.

If anybody mentioned the word "psychology," I thought mental illness. I looked it up. There are a whole slough of areas in this field. The part I am most interested in is the Greek root, "psyche"... meaning soul.

I took the Greek meanings of the words; *Meta* = beyond, *physical* = 3D, *Psyche* = soul, and *ology* = the study of. I would define it like this: *The study of the soul that is beyond the 3D world.* This is a very simple definition, that works for me.

Why did I choose metaphysical psychology? Metaphysical teachings include a collection of "New-Age" concepts, Ageless Wisdom, divine energies, and cosmic support..

Metaphysics also teaches us how to harness and apply these forces that are within us. Metaphysics teaches us how to be "in tune" with nature and with the divine plan of the universe.

God gave man the right to choose, and this privilege should not be taken away. There is the freedom from the religious dogma. We are told not to take "their" word for any-

Surviving MRSA

thing. It is up to us, with our connection with "the source," to determine what "is true" for us. The soul loves freedom. If man or the soul were to be caged, it would be a violation to the natural order of things.

The psychology portion (study of the soul) fits with my quest. Man-made laws can, and are, manipulated by unscrupulous people. In the laws of our society, the innocent are often made to pay for the crimes of others.

Anything that would help to refine one's soul character, and expand one's knowledge, is beneficial. That is another reason for studying metaphysics. A student of metaphysics is equally comfortable studying the teachings of everything between Alchemy and Zen (which I have).

By exploring the various teachings, students of metaphysics, probe the core beliefs of the various religions. Going back to their source or Ageless Teachings. I am not limited to one set of beliefs. I am able to seek out and embrace those ancient teachings.

Dr Joseph Parazoo

Surviving MRSA

Dr Joseph Parazoo

References

Allen, Jane, "Stroke Therapy" April 2003;
Los Angeles Times LA, www.latimes.com

American Medical Association, www.web-health.com :
"Blood Tests: Complete Blood Count" July 2005

Bain, Lisa, MD, "Managing MS Through Rehabilitation 2005;
National MS Society, www.nationalmssociety.org

Bliss, David P. Jr, MD, "Necrotizing fasciitis after Plastibell circumcision" September 1997;
Journal of Pediatrics, Children's Hospital & Medical Center, University of Washington, Seattle

Center for Disease Control and Prevention Atlanta, GA, www.cdc.gov: "Group A Streptococcal (GAS) Disease— Necrotizing Fasciitis" October 2005; "Group A Streptococcal (GAS) Disease— Strep Throat" August 2005

Cronin, Colleen, "Necrotizing Fasciitis (Flesh-Eating Bacteria)" British Columbia Ministry of Health Services, www.bchealthguide.org

Davies, H Dele, MD, MSc, June 2001; "Flesh-eating disease: A note on Necrotizing fasciitis": Pulsus Group Inc

DeBakey, Michael, MD, "Skin Grafts" 2005; Baylor College, Houston, Texas, www.baylor.vasculardomain.com :

Surviving MRSA

DHPE; Group B Streptococcus www.dhpe.org :

Eidelson, Stewart, MD, "Drop Foot and Steppage Gait" August 2003; Spine Universe, www.spineuniverse.com

Farlander "Streptococcus Pyogenes—Killer Flesh-eating Bacteria" February 2003: British Broadcasting Corporation www.bbc.co.uk

Gerritsen, Tess, *Life Support* 1997; Pocket Books New York

Havill, Sonya, MD, "Skin Grafting", 2002; DermNet, www.dermnetnz.org : Hamilton, New Zealand

Health-Care Net, www.health-cares.net: "Necrotizing Fasciitis" 2005

Hoe, Nancy, "Rapid Molecular Genetic Subtyping of Serotype M1 Group A Streptococcus Strains" April 1999; Baylor College of Medicine, Houston, Texas, www.cdc.gov/ncidod/EID/vol5no2/hoe.htm

Koontz, Dean, *Phantoms* 1983; GP Putnam's Sons, New York

Maynor, Michael, MD; WebMD www.emedicine.com :

"Necrotizing Fasciitis" December 2006

Mckern, Leo, "MRSA" April 2004: British Broadcasting Corporation www.bbc.co.uk

Mesa, Ruben MD, "High White Blood Cell Count" September

Dr Joseph Parazoo

2006; Mayo Foundation for Medical Education and Research, www.mayoclinic.com :

Miller, Loren G., M.D., M.P.H., "Necrotizing Fasciitis Caused by Community-Associated Methicillin-Resistant

MRSA Questions.. www.mrsaquestions.com

Staphylococcus aureus in Los Angeles" April 2005:
The New England Journal of Medicine,
www.content.nejm.org

Musher, Daniel, "Trends in Bacteremic Infection Due to Streptococcus pyogenes" February 1996; Veterans Affairs Medical Center, Houston, Texas

National Institute of Health www.niaid.nih.gov : "Group A Streptococcal Infections" November 2005

National Institute of Health: www.raredisease.info.nih.gov/asp/diseases/diseaseinfo.asp

National Necrotizing Fasciitis Foundation, www.nnff.org: "What is NF" August 2003

Nemours Foundation, www.kidshealth.org: "Seizures" October 2006

Neurology Channel, www.neurologychannel.com: "Epilepsy/Seizures" 2007

New York State Department of Health, "Streptococcal Infections"; June 2004

Surviving MRSA

Moore, Cassi; "NF Survivor" January 2004: www.nnff.org

Providence Health & Services, www.providence.org : "Mother Joseph of the Sacred Heart: Pioneer, Leader, Woman of Faith"

Public Health Agency of Canada, www.phac-aspc.gc.ca:

"Necrotizing Fasciitis/Myositis" April 1999

Public Health Seattle & King County, "Group A Strep

Necrotizing fasciitis (NF) Fact Sheet," April 2006: Seattle, Washington

Santora, Thomas, MD; WebMD, www.emedicine.com:

"Fournier Gangrene" Sheps, Sheldon, MD; "Gangrene" June 2006: Mayo Foundation, www.MayoClinic.com

Stevens, Dennis L., PhD, MD, "Streptococcal Toxic-Shock Syndrome" September 1995: University of Washington

School of Medicine, Seattle, Washington (www.cdc.gov/ncidod/EID/vol1no3/stevens.htm)

The Lee Spark NF Foundation, www.nfsuk.org.uk: "Septic Shock" 1999

University of Kentucky, agripedia www.uky.edu "Septicemic Plague" 1999

Dr Joseph Parazoo

US National Library of Medicine: "Gangrene"
www.nlm.nih.gov/medlineplus, Bethesda, MD

Wener, Kenneth, MD, "Necrotizing soft tissue infection,"
www.nlm.nih.gov/medlineplus Bethesda, MD

Wikipedia, www.en.wikipedia.org: Various words throughout.

Surviving MRSA

Dr Joseph Parazoo

About the Author

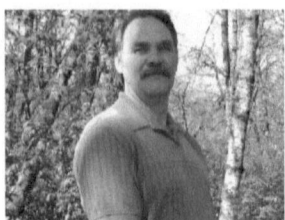

I have been married since 1978 to a wonderful soul, Kim.

We have 2 children and 3 grandchildren.

Early in 2005, Kim contracted what they call "necrotizing fasciitis" or "flesh eating bacteria." This caused me to have a very profound spiritual "experience." I have been on a "journey back home" ever since.

I have dedicated my life to the Spirit of the Universe - known as God, Oneness, All That Is, as well as many other names.

I also want to share my knowledge, gifts, and spirit with as many people as I can. Besides writing a couple of books, I record guided meditation, and provide healing as a Reiki Master. Please visit my website for more information.

I received a Doctor's degree in Metaphysical Psychology from the University of Sedona of Arizona, mainly for personal growth.

Website – http://joeparazoo.com

Surviving MRSA

Awakening to a New Consciousness

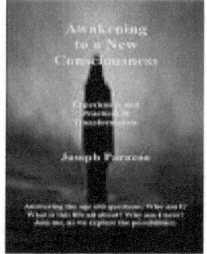

The application of metaphysical principles assists the acceleration of one's evolution. This takes us on a quantum leap to a higher level of knowledge and spiritual consciousness. Just to "know" is not enough. We have to practice and apply what we know.

When we work these principles in harmony with the cosmic laws, it empowers us with tools to achieve a successful and fulfilled life.

Maybe someday, somehow that spark that lives down deep, in the recesses of the "heaven within" residing in the inner chamber of the heart, will ignite. Causing you to start your quest through the various

Esoteric teachings available throughout the world. Answering the age old questions. Who am I? What is this life about? Why am I here? Starting your search inward. Join me, as we explore the possibilities.

Joseph Parazoo -- ISBN: 1-4382-2422-2

Dr Joseph Parazoo

Ancient Spiritual Exercises - Revealed

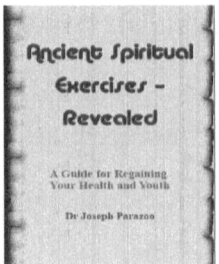

During my study of various religions, I have re-discovered or uncovered several exercises that have been kept secret for many years. These exercises have been used by monks, yogis, mystics, and enlightened ones for centuries.

Each of these exercises were designed for a specific purpose. They became sacred teachings, being taught only to a select few.

These exercises are very powerful and were highly prized. Many of these practices have been lost or forgotten because of this secrecy. Part of the secrecy was because of the punishment that was handed out for doing these exercises – usually death.

This book will explain the purpose behind the practices. It will walk you through each exercise – step-by-step. By properly following these instructions -- you will regain your health and vitality. With continued practice – you will recover your youthful looks.

Joseph Parazoo ISBN: 144042229X